LOVE WHAT YOU EAT:
CHOOSING FOODS THAT
WILL CHANGE YOUR LIFE

NICHOLETTE M. MARTIN, MD, HC

authorHOUSE®

AuthorHouse™ LLC
1663 Liberty Drive
Bloomington, IN 47403
www.authorhouse.com
Phone: 1-800-839-8640

Published by AuthorHouse   09/02/2014

ISBN: 978-1-4969-3562-5 (sc)
ISBN: 978-1-4969-3549-6 (e)

Library of Congress Control Number: 2014915048

TABLE OF CONTENTS

ACKNOWLEDGMENTS

This book would not have been possible without the help and support of many. First I thank God for giving me the insight to write *Love What You Eat*, and for sustaining me with the idea for over five years. Special thanks to my parents who have always been the "wind beneath my wings." To Dwayne for his patience and support and (slightly) unbiased review. To Jay and Suzanne for their guidance and direction. And last but not least, to Oso and Oslo (my Rottweilers), for always reminding me of what's really important - good food, lots of sleep and having some fun every day!

PREFACE

My motivation for writing this book is both personal and professional. Being raised in the Midwest meant I grew up on a diet containing a lot of meat and potatoes, with veggies on the side. Because I was always athletic, I could eat whatever I wanted. In my teens, pizza and ice cream was my favorite meal! In my twenties I began to have trouble tolerating my "favorite meal." I experienced nausea, bloating... the works. I found out I was lactose intolerant, so dairy was now my enemy! After a few years of lactose-free milk and lactose pills, I decided to listen to my body. It was saying "no mas" to dairy and that was that. I converted to soy products, and began to feel much better.

Fast forward thirty years. I began to read about Greek yogurt. Because of the way it's processed, some people with lactose intolerance are able to eat it. It turned out that I was one of those people... sort of. Overjoyed with this new found freedom, I began to eat it EVERY DAY. I had side effects, but they were mild, so I tried to ignore them. I began to get some joint stiffness and felt sluggish, but continued exercising and loving my yogurt. Then one day, BAM!!! A routine gynecological exam revealed some abnormalities. This required a uterine biopsy, and then another. I had cancer. What, me??? Me, the health nut, gym rat and yoga lover had cancer?? I NEVER saw that coming.

As I sat at home recuperating from a total hysterectomy, I continued to wonder: Was it due to my intake of dairy after thirty years (see *The China Study* by Thomas M. Campbell and T. Colin Campbell)? Was it due to hormones, or was it genetics? Was it all three working against me, or none of the above? It's impossible to point to one factor as the cause of most cancers. But there are a few things I know for sure: how truly blessed I am to have my life and health and, that I'm meant to help others figure out what makes them healthy and keeps them on their path to a long, fulfilling life.

INTRODUCTION

As a physician specializing in pain management, I see my patients struggling with weight issues every day. Although many of them ask for information about healthy foods, they have trouble following a specific program or sticking to a "diet." Some of them think they would have to eat only organic foods or become vegans. Ultimately they get frustrated and after a very short amount of time, just give up. I want to show my patients and anyone else who needs help finding a balanced, appealing and easy to manage plan for eating healthy foods that there is ANOTHER WAY.

Chances are that if you have picked up this book, you are overweight and concerned about your health. You may have the symptoms of metabolic syndrome: high blood pressure, high cholesterol, excessively large abdominal girth and/or adult onset diabetes. You may know that these four conditions lead to an increased possibility of stroke, heart attack and subsequent death. Your spouse or parent or child may have expressed concern about your health. Your doctor has likely counseled you to lose weight and has gone over the various life-threatening conditions you're dealing with because of your weight. You probably don't feel good or like the way you look – your clothes are uncomfortable, your joints are painful, you get winded climbing a small flight of stairs, you don't fit into airplane seats or movie theater seats, your life is feeling more and more circumscribed and you feel ashamed and even terrified that you have put your life in jeopardy.

Perhaps you have tried to diet. Perhaps you have tried the Atkins or South Beach or Jenny Craig approaches to weight loss. Maybe you've attended Weight Watcher's meetings and maybe you've successfully lost weight as a result of adhering to one or more of these diet plans. Maybe you have lost weight many times, only to gain it back each and every time. Perhaps you have adopted a vegan or vegetarian diet or ascribed to an Ayurvedic, macrobiotic or raw foods approach to weight loss. There may have been periods in your life when, as a result of dieting, you have been at a weight that felt good. Maybe you threw out your "fat clothes" and vowed that you'd never gain the weight back. You were valiant in your efforts to maintain your diet, but the discipline, the tedium, the time commitment, the restrictions, and the absolute focus it took to stay on your diet began to wear you out. You cheated, you hid, you denied, you beat yourself up and eventually you gained all the weight back, and more.

You are not overweight because you lack discipline, are lazy or irresponsible. There are a number of reasons why you are overweight and they're not all your fault. You have been misled and manipulated by the food manufacturing companies that produce most of what you find in grocery stores. This is why there is an "obesity epidemic" in the United States. In this book, I'll talk about what ingredients are really in processed foods, including so-called healthy choices, many of which are so high in sodium, that you are getting at least three or four times the daily recommended amount in one "healthy" serving. I will encourage you to pay attention to what you are eating, to read the labels on your processed foods and become aware of the ingredients that are not good for you. I know many of you think you're doing the right thing, and you want to do the right thing, but you're frustrated and don't know why you're still gaining weight even when you are choosing foods that claim to be healthy and low in fat, cholesterol and calories.

Most of the processed foods you eat, when broken down by the body, are stored as fat. As your fat cells get fatter, the receptor sites on the cells stretch so insulin (the hormone that allows you to use sugar for energy) can no longer bond to those sites, which causes the excess sugar to stay in your bloodstream rather than being processed and utilized as energy by your body. The excess sugar in your bloodstream is what causes diabetes. Eating processed foods can also increase the "bad" cholesterol in your bloodstream which leads to plaque in the arteries. Plaque creates blockages in the arteries which increase blood pressure and can ultimately result in stroke or heart attack.

While food is unequivocally the main contributing factor in the obesity epidemic, I cannot ignore the other contributing factors, the most damaging of which is lack of exercise in part due to our technology driven culture – a culture that encourages us to sit for hours in front of a computer or television screen. I will not provide an exercise plan in this book, as I have chosen to focus almost exclusively on diet and nutrition, but I will say that if you can just walk, even five minutes a day (to start), you will eventually see a difference in muscle tone, aerobic capacity and energy level, which will ultimately help you lose weight, feel better and become healthier.

I will, however, devote a chapter in this book to what is referred to as "Primary Foods." These are the psychological reasons behind why you eat to excess and why you eat even when you are not hungry. Most people generally don't think about "Primary Foods" – they think, "I'm overweight because my mother was overweight, it's genetic or I eat a lot and I eat junk." Well why do you eat a lot? Are you hungry? Why do you go for comfort food? Why is it called comfort food? Why do you go for mac and cheese as opposed to a salad when you're feeling stressed or lonely or your heart has been broken?

I will help you identify the various areas - finances, career, spirituality, relationships, health and physical activity - that may be affecting your psychological state to the extent that you are sabotaging your health by eating food you know is bad for you. This information will help you become aware of your traumas, patterns and triggers, which will help you make healthier choices. Until you understand why you make the choices you do, it's going to be hard for you to convince yourself that you need to make different choices. By identifying the areas in your life that are causing you the emotional pain and stress that you have been stuffing down by overeating and/or indulging in junk food, you will have the power to make positive changes. When you become clear about what is motivating you to consume three doughnuts and a Pepsi for breakfast, or inhale a tub of ice cream at ten o'clock at night, you will have the information you need to seek the kind of support that will be most healing for you. It may be psychological or spiritual counseling, financial or professional advice, a 12-Step program or support group, or simply a trusted friend or family member who is willing to be your sounding board and advocate.

This is NOT a diet book! My intention in writing this book, is to provide you with a different approach to creating and maintaining a healthy body, positive mind-set and fulfilling life. I will provide you with information about the various popular diets that are being promoted as cure-alls for permanent weight loss and improved health. I will educate you about the foods you eat and how they affect your body inside and out. I will provide you with healthy and appealing alternatives to the junk food you think you cannot live without, and I will encourage you to find ways to support yourself in your quest for greater health and well-being. I intend to promote easy, practical and inexpensive lifestyle changes that may ultimately result in permanent weight loss and greatly improved health.

The approach I am offering to better health and weight loss is not something you do for six weeks, and then abandon for your old habits. My approach is designed to provide long-term, sustainable results. Strict diets and maintenance plans have generally not been shown to work in the long run. I am proposing small changes that create lasting results. If you have picked up this book, I assume you are willing to take responsibility for your health and are open to learning about how your body works and what simple, common sense steps you can take to create and support YOUR best possible life. You are not the only one who suffers when you are overweight and unhappy. Your friends and family suffer with you.

I am a physician who has been working with chronic pain patients for over eighteen years. Many of my patients struggle with obesity. I became interested in nutrition and diet as a way to provide extra support for these particular patients. It is my dream to reach out to those of you who are willing to take responsibility for your health, and are open to making small, but meaningful changes in your lifestyle. I want to help you before you get to the point where you need my services as a pain doctor!

I am approaching dieting and health from a doctor's point of view. I am motivated by my doctor's instinct to help other people, which is supported by my upbringing and nurtured by my spiritual beliefs. It is my mission to help you feel better by encouraging you to make the lifestyle and dietary changes that will improve your health and give you the energy to pursue your dreams. These are the dreams that are often left to languish and ultimately die when you suffer from obesity and the attendant debilitating health issues. I want to give you back your life, to help you help yourself!

At the end of the day, if you don't feel good, you may ask yourself why you bother to get up in the morning or why you even exist at all. I acknowledge that there are a lot of factors that influence these kinds of despairing thoughts, but what you eat and how you choose to nourish your body, has a powerful impact on how you feel and what you think. Your diet is a great place to begin making the changes that will eventually help you feel better and allow you to start dreaming about the true purpose of your life.

If you can have a better day today than you did yesterday, and a better day tomorrow, wouldn't it be better for your family, your kids, and for your existence? EVERYONE needs to find his or her purpose and get about the business of fulfilling it, and you can't do that if you're stuck in a rut. We all struggle. I want to help you take the next step. I don't want to drag you, but I will support you. I'm here to help you discover how much better you can feel and how much better you can be. How cool would it be to feel good <u>and</u> look good? With a few non-diet changes to your diet, it really can happen. What if this book could change your life? Would you want to read it? I hope your answer is a resounding yes!

EAT WHAT YOU LOVE, LOVE WHAT YOU EAT!

Chapter One

THE MYSTERIOUS WAYS OF THE FOOD INDUSTRY

I have used the word, "mysterious," in the title of this chapter for a reason. In my experience, I have found that there is a lot of confusion about which foods are actually healthy and what qualities constitute a healthy food product. If a packaged food product is labeled, "Zero Trans-Fats," "Gluten-Free," "Non-Fat" or "Heart-Healthy," doesn't that make it a healthy choice? How many grams of sugar, sodium and fat are acceptable anyway? Aren't foods with added vitamins and minerals healthy? And what are all those other unpronounceable ingredients? What the heck is a GMO and why is it bad, or is it? It may be obvious that sugar encrusted cereals are not a healthy choice, but what about the cereals that claim to lower cholesterol levels? Isn't that a good thing?

American consumers are generally savvy, but there are so many false claims made in advertising campaigns for food products, and there are so many conflicting declarations from "experts" about what is healthy and what is not, that it's almost impossible to figure out what to eat to maintain good health, never mind what to eat to actually cure disease. It's easy to understand why big food companies want to appeal to your best impulses or your genuine health concerns by claiming that their foods are healthy; but, isn't it illegal to misrepresent their products and aren't there government regulations in place to keep those companies honest? If the FDA (Food and Drug Administration) and the USDA (United States Department of Agriculture) approve of a product or advocate the consumption of a certain kind of food, doesn't that mean it's healthy?

Politics of Food

The United States Department of Agriculture (USDA), which is a federal regulatory agency, does in fact offer Dietary Guidelines to the general public. Older guidelines used a Food Pyramid, which was first introduced to the public in 1992 and then updated in 2005. The original Pyramid orders the food groups horizontally, with the largest group at the base of the Pyramid being the grains group: bread, rice, pasta and cereal. The second level up represents vegetables and fruit. The third level represents protein and dairy. The protein group includes meat, poultry, fish, dried beans, nuts and eggs, and the dairy group includes cheese, yogurt and milk. The top of the Pyramid represents fats, oils and sweets.

In 2005, the Pyramid was redesigned so that the food groups were represented by vertical bands of color, each delineating one of the food groups. The grains, vegetables and milk groups are about equal and altogether represent 73% of the total. Fruits represent 15%, meats and beans represent 10%, and oils represent 2%. Currently, the guidelines come in the form of something called: MyPlate (http://www.choosemyplate.gov/), which was introduced in 2011. The MyPlate website includes information about nutrition as well as a diagram of a plate of food and a cup. The plate is separated into four (almost equal) sections that delineate four separate food groups: fruits, vegetables, grains and protein, with the cup representing dairy.

The USDA nutritional guidelines are taught in public schools, and used as a template for what gets served in public schools, to the military and in other government funded institutions. Though you may or may not be familiar with the guidelines, they are extremely influential and determine what a lot of Americans, particularly school children are eating.

Unfortunately, the USDA's Dietary Guidelines are a questionable resource. Some of the recommendations may be quite good, but the federal regulatory agencies have rightly been accused of pandering to the huge, multi-national food corporations that they are meant to be monitoring. This conflict of interest on the part of the government means that the guidelines reflect the best interests of the food industry, not the best interests of the American people. When the first Food Pyramid was proposed in 1991, the meat and dairy industries protested because they felt their products weren't given enough space. It took a year for the USDA to negotiate with the meat and dairy industries to come up with a diagram everyone could agree on. "Let's face it; the 1991 USDA Food Pyramid is a political document, not a scientific one. It encourages people to eat a lot of everything. This advice certainly helps the food industry and the senators protecting their financial interests." (Joshua Rosenthal, *Integrative Nutrition*)

Food industry lobbyists have a huge influence in Washington, because the food industry generates trillions of dollars annually. For instance, lobbyists for the meat industries have successfully managed, time and again, to delay or halt the implementation of safety regulations that would require more extensive testing for E. coli and salmonella in beef and other meats. The meat industry will do anything in its power to prevent regulations that will cost them money, which can put the consumer in jeopardy. Senators and Congressmen from states with politically strong agricultural or meat producing businesses, will not risk angering those businesses for fear of losing elections. The food industry contributes huge amounts of money to political campaigns.

In fact, the food industry receives protection from the government in the form of food libel laws. Thirteen states have passed these laws. They differ from state to state, but essentially allow any food producer, processor or manufacturer in those states to sue anyone who criticizes their food product. You may remember the famous case in which Oprah Winfrey was sued by a group of Texas cattle ranchers for making a disparaging remark about hamburger on a show in which she was interviewing a former cattle rancher about mad-cow disease. She ultimately won, but only after spending as much as one million dollars on her defense!

Commercial Agriculture

The United States government has been subsidizing farmers since the 1920's. Originally this was intended to help farmers stay afloat by keeping their costs down and boosting sales of their low-priced products. As a result of these subsidies, there is now an enormous surplus of corn and soybeans grown every year. Because of this, corn and soybean meal is fed to factory farm animals (livestock raised in crowded, inhumane conditions in order to maximize production and minimize cost) and even farmed fish - none of whom are genetically designed to eat corn.

In the mid-1970's, in order to make use of this surplus corn, high-fructose corn syrup (which had been invented in the late '50's) was introduced into soft drinks and processed foods in the United States to take the place of white sugar, which was more expensive (and still is). High-fructose corn syrup also has the added advantage for the manufacturer of lengthening the shelf-life of the packaged food products to which it is added. The potential health risks of consuming high-fructose corn syrup is a hotly debated topic. There are those who feel it has significantly contributed to the obesity epidemic and all the diseases associated with obesity. Recently, some companies have replaced high-fructose corn syrup with sugar in some of their products. Nonetheless, it remains a substantial ingredient in hundreds if not thousands of processed, packaged, pre-prepared and fast food items.

As it turns out, 90% of surplus corn is now genetically modified, and 80% is grown from the Monsanto Company's patented genetically modified seeds. Monsanto is a multi-national, chemical and agricultural biotechnology corporation. GM (Genetically Modified) food is wildly controversial, as the long-term consequences of ingesting GM foods is not known. Those who manufacture GM crops claim they improve the crop by making it more resistant to destruction by pests, herbicides, drought, cold or disease. Many feel that GM crops have been allowed to proliferate without being adequately tested first due to lack of government regulation. Animal studies and anecdotal evidence in human responses and reactions have demonstrated that there may be health risks associated with eating GM foods, from allergic reactions and reproductive problems to liver damage and death.

Because farm subsidies have increasingly gone to corn and soybeans over the years, there is much less government money for other crops, keeping the cost of growing vegetables, fruit and other grains higher, a cost that is then passed on to the consumer. Another issue with American crops in general is that today's farming practices deplete the soil of nutritionally necessary vitamins and minerals which are not replaced with fertilizer. Because of this, non-organic vegetables and fruits are not as rich in life-sustaining nutrients as they once were. This means that if you rely on a more plant-based diet, you may not be getting all the nutrients you need to support optimal health. This is just another consequence of lack of over-sight by the governing bodies who are meant to be protecting our food supply.

Commercial Meat and Dairy

There are numerous ethical and health issues associated with eating meat and dairy in general and commercial meat and dairy in particular. Commercially raised farm animals - hogs, cattle, milk cows and chickens - are kept in over-crowded, filthy feedlots, concrete stalls, cages or large windowless sheds, where they stand or lie in their own manure day in and day out.

They are over-fed the cheaply produced GM corn and soybeans and injected with hormones to fatten them quickly. Then they are treated with antibiotics to kill the bacteria that the corn and soybean feed and unsanitary living conditions breed. Fattening the animals too quickly often makes it hard for them to stand or move, so larger animals like cattle are frequently beaten to get them to move. The brutal and inhumane treatment of farm animals also extends to the workers who tend to them and slaughter them. Slaughterhouse workers are covered in feces, blood and urine all day long and work like machines, completing one task over and over again. They frequently suffer from illnesses and injuries related to the dangerously unsanitary conditions, as well as repetitive strain injuries such as tendinitis, carpal tunnel syndrome and edema.

Producing truly safe meat can be costly, and the meat industry is known to fight any proposed legislation that would increase production costs or alert the consumer to the possibility that meat might be unsafe to eat. The truth is that because commercial farm animals stand in their own feces for the duration of their lives, their hides or feathers are coated in manure when they are brought to slaughter, so it is impossible to keep the manure out of the meat. This vastly increases the possibility of E. coli contamination. The runoff from factory farms periodically contaminates nearby crops which has caused over the years mass recalls of various vegetables (food that would not normally be exposed to contamination by bacteria like E. coli).

The environmental issues associated with factory farming are numerous and potentially devastating. Aside from the effects of runoff from the manure "lagoons," mentioned above, the untreated manure can contaminate groundwater, nearby streams, rivers and lakes and thus well water and other sources of drinking water. Communities adjacent to huge factory farm feedlots can suffer from air pollution as well as water pollution. The toxic gases emitted from large amounts of manure contain compounds such as ammonia and methane, which are poisonous and can cause allergic reactions, and more seriously, respiratory illnesses, such as asthma. Perhaps most disturbingly, the enormous amount of greenhouse gasses emitted from the vast quantities of manure generated by factory farms has been said to be contributing to global warming. "The methane releases from billions of imprisoned animals on factory farms are 70 times more damaging per ton to the earth's atmosphere than CO2." (http://ecowatch.com)

Commercial Food Industry

Most of us can agree that we love sugar, salt and fat: salt & vinegar potato chips, glazed donuts, ice cream, cookies, and fast food burgers with french fries. The list could go on and on. Even those of us who generally try to eat healthy food, occasionally indulge in something we might consider to be a guilty pleasure, or a well-earned treat, or compensation for a particularly bad day or more typically a broken heart. There is no one who understands this better than the food industry giants like Nestle, Kraft, General Mills, Kellogg and Hershey, just to name a few. These companies use science to determine exactly how much sugar, salt and fat will create the state they refer to as the "bliss point." This is the feeling that makes it impossible to eat just one (or three, or twenty) potato chips or cookie. The food industry knows how to stimulate your taste buds and more importantly, your brain, so you literally become addicted to the food they're selling. Make no mistake, they know what they're doing and they do it deliberately, in spite of evidence that their food is contributing to the declining health of a large number of Americans, as well as many people around the world who have adopted a more American-style diet.

Not only are the big food companies designing products that we literally can't resist, they refuse to take any responsibility for the obesity epidemic their products contribute to. And they continue to overtly target children in their ad campaigns. Even if you have barely paid attention to the news in the last twenty years, you have had to notice that more and more children are suffering from obesity and early-onset type 2 diabetes.The food companies know that children are particularly vulnerable to marketing and they are devising ever more insidious ways to get them to eat their food products. Adults who are concerned with weight and health, should not be deceived by the food industry's promotion of "healthy," packaged and pre-prepared, processed food products. Foods that are billed as "low-fat," very often have more sugar and salt added to make up for the flavor lost by reducing fat. Cereals that claim to contain healthy "whole grains," more often than not contain *processed* whole grains. Processed whole grains elevate blood sugar levels, real whole grains generally do not. So the moral of the story: The food industry is not your friend!

One of the most deceptive and damaging aspects of all processed food is that it is calorie dense and nutrient poor. In other words, you have to eat more processed food than real, whole, nutrient rich food to feel full and fully satiated. The calories add up, while you eat more and more food trying to get the nutrients your body craves, but will never get from processed food. That's why you want to eat again soon after finishing off a processed food meal.

Obesity Epidemic

Which brings me to the obesity epidemic in the United States. The U.S. has the distinction of being the second fattest country in the entire world! About one third of the population of the US over twenty years old is considered obese and almost three quarters of the population over twenty is considered overweight if you include those who are obese. More upsetting still is the fact that almost one third of children and adolescents in the U.S. have been determined to be overweight or obese.

The American Medical Association defines obesity as a disease and a person is considered obese if his or her Body Mass Index (BMI) is 30 or higher. BMI is used as an approximate measurement of body fat and is determined by calculating height versus weight. See the chart below to determine your approximate BMI:

HEIGHT	WEIGHT															
	100	110	120	130	140	150	160	170	180	190	200	210	220	230	240	250
5'0"	20	21	23	25	27	29	31	33	35	37	39	41	43	45	47	49
5'1"	19	21	23	25	26	28	30	32	34	36	38	40	42	43	45	47
5'2"	18	20	22	24	26	27	29	31	33	35	37	38	40	42	44	46
5'3"	18	19	21	23	25	27	28	30	32	34	35	37	39	41	43	44
5'4"	17	19	21	22	24	26	27	29	31	33	34	36	38	39	41	43
5'5"	17	18	20	22	23	25	27	28	30	32	33	35	37	38	40	42
5'6"	16	18	19	21	23	24	26	27	29	31	32	34	36	37	39	40
5'7"	16	17	19	20	22	23	25	27	28	30	31	33	34	36	38	39
5'8"	15	17	18	20	21	23	24	26	27	29	30	32	33	35	36	38
5'9"	15	16	18	19	21	22	24	25	27	28	30	31	32	34	35	37
5'10"	14	16	17	19	20	22	23	24	26	27	29	30	32	33	34	36
5'11"	14	15	17	18	20	21	22	24	25	26	27	28	30	32	33	35
6'0"	14	15	16	18	19	20	22	23	24	26	27	28	30	31	33	34
6'1"	13	15	16	17	18	20	21	22	24	25	26	28	29	30	32	33
6'2"	13	14	15	17	18	19	21	22	23	24	26	27	28	30	31	32
6'3"	12	14	15	16	17	19	20	21	22	24	25	26	27	29	30	31
6'4"	12	13	15	16	17	18	19	21	22	23	24	26	27	28	29	30

The health issues associated with obesity are heart disease, heart attack, metabolic syndrome, diabetes, cancer, high blood pressure, stroke, allergies, sleep apnea, asthma, joint problems, back problems, osteoarthritis, gallstones, gall bladder disease, liver disease, menstrual problems, infertility and psychological problems, such as depression and social anxiety. Being obese is no fun and ultimately life threatening. Although obesity itself is considered a disease, it is also considered to be a "leading preventable cause of death worldwide." (http://en.wikipedia. org/wiki/Obesity)

If obesity is thought of as a leading preventable cause of death it could also be considered a leading preventable cause of the illnesses listed above. Yes, the food industry has seduced the public with misleading information and created irresistible products that have made Americans and others around the world fat. But why has obesity become an epidemic and why are the numbers of obese children and adults increasing every year? It is easy to point the finger at the food industry and rail against the government for not protecting its citizens. Certainly economic factors have played a crucial role, but in the end, it is each individual's responsibility to take care of his or her body, and each parent's job to nurture and care for his or her child. We have created a culture that worships speed and demands convenience, and in the process we have sacrificed our quality of life. IT MAKES NO SENSE TO PAY LESS FOR FAST FOOD, ONLY TO PAY MORE FOR PRESCRIPTION DRUGS AND MEDICAL CARE. It makes no sense to opt for convenience and speed in the short term, only to sacrifice mobility and energy in the long term.

Self-responsibility

We can no longer afford to be the victims of industries that do not have our best interests at heart. We can no longer afford to sacrifice our health for cheap or convenient food. We must become educated and we must find reasonable alternatives to the donut and soda breakfast, drive-through burger and Frappuccino lunch, and microwave dinner. Identifying foods for yourself and your family that are nutritious, tasty and easy to prepare, is the first step to change. And every journey begins with the FIRST STEP! It may take a shift in consciousness, but a healthy, active and agile body, a clear, positive mind, a high-level of energy and the ability to experience life more fully are worth the small amount of effort it will take to make the change.

Chapter Two

WHY IT MATTERS WHAT YOU EAT:

How Food Affects Your Body Inside and Out

There are a lot of things that can affect your health, but what you put IN your body is one of the most important. Many illnesses can be caused and cured by diet alone. Certain foods that cause inflammation (in joints, tissues etc...) also cause chronic disease conditions (diabetes, heart disease, arthritis and even some auto-immune diseases). These foods are what you would expect: trans fats, white sugar and white flour products. These foods cause free radical formation (one of the major causes of cancer), and other caustic substances to be produced in the body, leading to internal damage. On the other hand, healthy, ANTI-inflammatory foods that prevent free radical formation (and therefore disease) include: wild-caught fish; lean organic and free-range meats; raw nuts; fresh, organic leafy greens and veggies; fresh fruit; certain organic coffees and green teas; good DARK chocolate; RED wine; garlic and olive oil.

If we're paying attention, we can all describe how different foods and beverages make us feel. There are a whole range of sensations and emotions we experience during and after eating, from pleasantly full, happy, satisfied and energized, to bloated, nauseated, drained, sleepy and/or irritable. Unfortunately, our eating habits are often so entrenched and unconscious, that we may not fully register how we actually feel - good or bad - after eating, and we most probably do not think about how the food we're eating affects our organs and tissues. This chapter will give you a good idea of how the food you're eating on a regular basis is impacting your body, inside and out. This information is meant to empower you by giving you the impetus to consider more carefully the food you choose to put in your body. Keeping your body healthy and happy is your responsibility... After all, it's the only body you've got!

THE IMPACT OF FOOD ON YOUR ORGANS, GLANDS AND TISSUES:

Heart

The human heart is located in the center of the chest, behind the breastbone, and tilts slightly to the left. It is approximately the size of a large fist and weighs, on the average, eleven ounces. The heart is an organ that acts as a muscular pump. Through rhythmic contractions, the heart moves blood to all parts of the body via a series of blood vessels know as arteries, veins and capillaries. Blood supplies essential nutrients and other vital substances like hormones and oxygen to the cells. It also carries away waste from the cells, which is eventually excreted through lungs, sweat, urine and feces.

The heart is comprised of three layers and divided into four chambers. The septum, a muscular wall, separates the right and left sides of the heart, which have different functions. The right side of the heart fills up with deoxygenated blood coming from the body and pushes it into the lungs where it is replenished with oxygen before it is recirculated back into the left side of the heart, and then pumped back into the body, where it provides life-giving oxygen to the cells. A healthy, adult human heart (at rest) beats sixty to seventy times per minute, and is able to beat due to a specialized group of cells in the heart (a natural pacemaker) that have the ability to generate electrical activity.

As you can imagine, this amazing organ is affected by what you eat and drink. There are many heart conditions that have been proven to be the result of an unhealthy, nutrient deficient diet. In fact, many cardiovascular diseases (an umbrella term for all diseases of the heart and blood vessels), can be attributed to the over-consumption of trans fats, sugar, salt and refined carbohydrates, all the ingredients you find in processed foods of all kinds: pre-prepared, packaged and fast foods. Did you know that cardiovascular disease is the cause of half of all the deaths in the United States each year and is the primary cause of death in adults?

Recently there have been new studies showing that sugar (including high fructose corn syrup and all other forms of *refined* sugar) and refined carbohydrates (such as white flour) are more detrimental to heart health than saturated fats and foods with a high cholesterol content, which have been demonized for years as the major contributing causes of heart disease. As I've said before, and will probably say again... and again, one of the main ingredients in almost all processed food is SUGAR! Sugar causes inflammation in the arteries, which can then trigger a cascade of events which will eventually lead to arterial blockage and possible heart attack and/or stroke.

Although sugar is one of the main culprits of inflammation in the body, trans fats (partially hydrogenated oils) are also extremely damaging and have been proven to cause inflammation and plaque build-up in the arteries, which can lead to heart attack. Trans fats have been under severe scrutiny lately and may be banned altogether at some point in the (hopefully near) future. As of this moment, the United States Food and Drug Administration (FDA) requires food manufacturers to list the amount of trans fats in their packaged products on the nutritional content labels, BUT companies that sell fast foods do not have to disclose the amount of trans fats in their products!

The *real* heart healthy foods are: fresh fruits and vegetables; high fiber foods such as whole grains and beans; healthy fats such as olive oil and walnut oil; foods that contain healthy fats, such as avocados and raw nuts; and foods that are high in omega-3 fatty acids, such as salmon and tuna. Foods with white fleshy centers, like apples, pears and cucumbers can lower your risk of stroke. According to the American Heart Association, almost 52 % lower! All of these foods help to reduce inflammation in the body and provide nutrients that reduce LDL ("bad" cholesterol) and boost HDL ("good" cholesterol), as well as reduce triglycerides (a type of fat found in the blood that in high amounts has been linked to heart disease and heart attack).

You may be happy to know that there is a specific candy that can be GOOD for your heart: CHOCOLATE. Yes, it's true, and I'm not just saying it because I'm a chocoholic from way back. In the 1700's cocoa was used to treat chest pain. Even though it can be on the side of "bad for you," chocolate has some real benefits. Studies have shown it can LOWER blood pressure, and decrease the risk of heart disease and strokes. It's the powerful anti-oxidant component that does the trick. Dark chocolate (70-80 %) has up to three times more anti-oxidants than milk chocolate. (White chocolate is no help at all!) Now let's not get crazy with this. It needs to be low in sugar as well. I'm not talking about a daily bag of M&Ms, but a couple of pieces of premium dark chocolate. Have this treat with 1-2 six ounce glasses of RED wine (more flavonoids to help protect the artery walls and boost HDL) as the perfect end to the perfect day! Your heart will thank you for it.

Brain

Although the adult human brain weighs only about three pounds, it uses twenty percent of the oxygen you inhale and twenty percent of the energy you consume through food and drink. It is an extremely complex organ and the hub of the central nervous system. The central nervous system controls every aspect of your life and your relationship with your environment. The brain receives information about the environment through nerves located in every part of the body. The nerves send information via chemical signals and electrical impulses to the brain through the spinal cord. The brain then processes the information and sends instructions back to the body through the spinal cord and nerves, thus dictating both conscious and unconscious behavioral responses and reactions to stimuli.

The brain itself is comprised of three main areas: the forebrain, midbrain and hindbrain and is divided down the middle into right and left hemispheres. The forebrain contains the cerebrum or cortex, which is the largest part of the brain and is divided into four "lobes." The lobes are responsible for higher brain functions such as thinking, reasoning, movement, memory, speech, visual and auditory perception, problem solving and emotions. The rest of the brain is responsible for everything from regulating movement and coordination to breathing and keeping the heart beating.

Because the brain uses twenty percent of the energy you consume through eating and drinking, what you consume has a profound effect on the function of the brain and by extension, the feelings you have, the behaviors you exhibit, the conscious responses and unconscious reactions you have, the choices you make and the automatic functions of the body. The brain is why we love salty, sweet, fatty food. It is in essence the reason we find those foods irresistible, delicious, addictive, comforting and emotionally satisfying. The brain tells us we love foods that are bad for us, but the brain, like every other part of the body, can only handle heavily processed foods that contain excessive amounts of trans fats, refined sugars, refined carbohydrates and salt, for so long before it and the entire central nervous system starts reacting.

Pigging out on half a bag of Pepperidge Farm cookies or sucking down a large, vanilla Frappuccino may make you feel "high," even energized and happy, but all too soon you will crash and burn, and very likely feel worse than you did before you indulged. The irritability and lethargy you experience as a result of a sugar crash are the short-term effects of ingesting too much sugar at one time. The long-term effects of excessive consumption of sugar are depression, impaired memory and cognitive function, as well as difficulty concentrating, which can cause difficulties learning. Sugar isn't the only substance that can impair brain function. There is current evidence suggesting that trans fats can interfere with the brain's ability to send messages to the body, which can result in anxiety, depression, lowering of cognitive ability, memory impairment and eventually degenerative diseases such as Alzheimer's.

The very best foods for brain function are foods that are high in anti-oxidants like blueberries, blackberries and raspberries; foods high in healthy fats like salmon, avocados, and extra-virgin olive oil; foods high in vitamin E like nuts, leafy greens, eggs, seeds and brown rice; and foods high in vitamin B, particularly B12, like salmon, tuna, shrimp, beef and yogurt. All these good brain-healthy foods can help stave off Alzheimer's disease and dementia, improve memory, lower blood pressure (which means increased blood flow to the brain), reduce inflammation and increase cognitive function.

Liver

The adult liver is about the size of a football, weighs approximately three pounds, is situated under the lower section of the rib cage and reaches across part of the abdominal cavity. The largest section of the liver sits to the right of the stomach and reaches down toward the right kidney. The gallbladder, pancreas and intestines sit beneath the liver and all work together to digest and absorb everything you put into your body. The liver's main jobs are to clean your blood and transform the nutrients and toxins you've ingested, so they can be used, stored or excreted. For example, when the liver processes carbohydrates, it extracts the glucose (sugar) and stores it as glycogen, which then becomes an emergency source of sugar, utilized as energy by the body when it's depleted. In addition, the liver produces a digestive juice called bile which helps in the digestion of fats. The liver also makes cholesterol (used by the body in the production of hormones) and proteins that help with blood clotting.

We all know that drinking alcohol in excess can be particularly bad for the liver. The liver has to work extra hard to process the toxins in alcohol, which means that it is distracted from its other functions leaving the body temporarily depleted of glucose (or energy). Glucose is essential for optimal brain functioning, which is why you feel hung-over (depleted, mentally hazy and ill), in the morning after a night of drinking too much. The long-term effects of excessive drinking can lead to liver disease (fatty liver and cirrhosis) and ultimately death. Some of the early symptoms of liver disease are jaundice, vomiting, swelling of legs and feet, a distended abdomen from fluid retention and confusion.

Aside from alcohol, processed foods (filled with trans fats, sugar and salt) are the main cause of liver disease. More and more studies are showing that processed foods cause liver enzymes to rise (the first sign of potential liver disease), just as they do with excess alcohol consumption. Obesity is another factor in liver damage, and we know that eating processed food on a regular basis can significantly contribute to weight gain, and ultimately lead to obesity. Liver damage can develop into something referred to as fatty liver disease, in which the liver literally becomes clogged with fat, adversely affecting its function. If left untreated, and if the eating and/or drinking habits that caused it are not altered, fatty liver disease will eventually progress to cirrhosis of the liver, in which the liver cells are replaced by scar tissue. Cirrhosis almost always leads to liver failure and death.

Foods that are rich in sulfur are particularly good for the liver because they promote liver detoxification. Sulfur rich foods include eggs, onions and garlic, as well as cruciferous vegetables, such as cauliflower, Brussels sprouts, broccoli, cabbage and kale. The liver also thrives on fresh fruits and all other vegetables, particularly grapefruit, beets, leafy greens, avocados and lemons. To keep your liver healthy, happy and functioning properly, you must eat a balanced diet of fresh foods, including the vegetables and fruits listed above, as well as clean, lean protein, healthy fats such as extra-virgin olive oil, nuts, and high-fiber foods like whole grains and beans.

Pancreas

The pancreas is a five inch long glandular organ, with an oblong, flattish shape. It sits between your stomach and your spinal column and extends toward the duodenum (top of the small intestines). It is part of the digestive and endocrine systems. The endocrine system refers to all the glands in the body, whose job it is to manufacture hormones which control reproduction, sexual development, growth and metabolism.

The pancreas contributes to digestion by secreting pancreatic juices containing digestive enzymes, which join bile coming from the liver with the partially digested food from the stomach in the duodenum, where they mix to continue the digestive process of breaking down the food to be utilized by the body, stored for later use, or excreted through the release of feces, urine or sweat.

The pancreas also releases the hormones, insulin and glucagon, which aid in the regulation of sugar in the bloodstream. Insulin helps glucose (sugar) from the blood nourish the cells. When glucose moves from the blood into the cells, the blood sugar levels are lowered which stimulates the pancreas to make glucagon. Glucagon then causes the liver to release glucose (sugar) into the blood, raising the blood sugar levels back to normal. In this way, the pancreas functions to regulate and stabilize the level of sugar in your blood, which ultimately keeps your energy level stable. There is a saying in medicine that every surgical intern learns: "Eat when you can, sleep when you can, but DON'T mess with the pancreas!" This organ has a very important job to do, and it is very particular about how it's treated.

So, just imagine what happens to the pancreas when you overload your body with sugar? Eating abnormally large amounts of sugar (as you do when you eat processed food or drink sugary soda, or over-indulge in alcohol), puts tremendous stress on the pancreas. This stress has a cumulative effect, and over time, takes a toll on the ability of the pancreas to regulate blood sugar levels. If you feed your body excessive amounts of sugar day after day, your pancreas will eventually break down and cease to be able to properly regulate blood sugar levels, meaning that sugar will build up in the blood, blood sugar levels will rise and you will ultimately experience a condition referred to as metabolic syndrome which can lead to diabetes. The symptoms and larger implications of metabolic syndrome and diabetes are discussed in greater length at the end of this chapter.

There is also evidence to suggest that foods high in trans fats, saturated fats and refined flours are bad for the optimal functioning of the pancreas. Those foods have been proven in some cases to cause pancreatitis or inflammation of the pancreas. The pancreas becomes inflamed when the digestive enzymes in the pancreatic juices are released too early and attack the pancreas instead of being released into the intestines. This condition can be extremely painful and can result in death in certain instances.

The best foods for the health of your pancreas are whole foods, such as fresh veggies and fruits, whole grains, healthy oils and lean proteins. Stay away from processed foods of all kinds and especially avoid refined sugars and flours. If you have pancreatic issues, I advise you to stay away from alcohol. The sugar in alcohol has the same negative effect on the pancreas that refined sugar does and can cause pancreatitis.

Kidneys

You have two kidneys, which is a good thing in case you lose one... always a possibility if you mistreat your body. And although you can live a long healthy life with only one kidney, let's not test that theory right now! An adult kidney is approximately the size of a clenched fist, four to five inches in length, and shaped like a "kidney" bean. These vital organs are located in the upper rear of the abdominal cavity, in the middle of the back next to the back muscles, one on either side of the spine. The kidneys are responsible for excreting waste from the body, as well as regulating blood pressure, red blood cell levels, acid levels and water levels in the body. In the excretion of wastes, the kidneys process around two hundred quarts of blood to filter out approximately two quarts of waste material and water. The waste and unneeded water is transferred as urine to the bladder, where it is stored until it is eliminated through urination.

One of the main causes of kidney disease is diabetes, and type 2 diabetes is often the result of the over-consumption of processed foods, especially food with a high refined sugar or carbohydrate content. Diabetes causes the glucose (sugar) levels in the blood to become elevated. The excess glucose can then damage the blood vessels of the kidneys, which means that the damaged kidneys cannot effectively filter out toxins from the body. As a result of this, the toxins flood the body, causing swelling, nausea and vomiting, shortness of breath, trouble sleeping, muscle cramps in the legs, high blood pressure, fatigue and a feeling of weakness. Kidney disease can eventually lead to kidney failure, which is why some people with advanced cases of type 2 diabetes end up on dialysis.

If you want to keep your precious kidneys functioning as they should, you will adopt a diet high in the whole foods I have been recommending throughout this chapter – including a wide variety of fresh vegetables and fruits, whole grains and beans, nuts and seeds, healthy fats, and lean meats. And for goodness sake, DRINK WATER!

Colon

Located in the abdomen, the colon (also known as the large intestine), is approximately five to six feet long, with a diameter of about two and one half inches. It is connected to the small intestine at one end and the rectum at the other. It is made up of four sections: the ascending colon, the transverse colon, the descending colon and the sigmoid colon. The colon is one of the organs that makes up the digestive system and serves to extract water, electrolytes (salts), and minerals from partially digested food. The colon then pushes, through a process referred to as peristalsis (wave-like muscular contractions), the left-over waste material (stool) into the rectum where it is stored for expulsion out of the body through the anus during a bowel movement.

The colon contains many different types of beneficial bacteria that aid in breaking down the partially digested food that enters from the small intestine. The majority of your immune system is … yes, is in your colon. This beneficial bacteria also protects against the proliferation of harmful bacteria. A healthy colon will easily eliminate toxins from the body and will keep you feeling good and energetic. A compromised or diseased colon will release toxins back into the body through the liver and bloodstream, where they will cause the entire body to become diseased. Processed foods high in sugar and trans fats will, over time, begin to destroy the good bacteria in your colon, which can cause an over growth of yeast and other "bad bugs" that interfere with digestion. When bad bacteria, yeast, fungi and even parasites have taken up residence in your colon, you will often feel bloated, uncomfortable and gassy, and may experience allergies, vaginal yeast infections, acne, constipation and/or diarrhea.

This break down in your colon's ability to process and expel waste matter can eventually lead to very serious conditions such as irritable bowel syndrome, autoimmune diseases, ulcerative colitis and colorectal cancer. In order to protect your colon and your health in general, I recommend the same high-fiber, whole foods diet I have been recommending all along. To prevent or correct health issues related to the colon, be sure to eat high-fiber foods that contain both soluble and insoluble fiber such as oatmeal, lentils, apples, nuts, flaxseeds and beans. Foods that contain probiotics such as plain yogurt and fermented foods like sauerkraut and miso will help prevent yeast over-growth and keep the good bacteria in the gut happy. Last but not least, drink plenty of water to keep everything moving!

Muscles

Muscles are a complex system of soft tissues that allow the body to move. Of the more than six hundred muscles in your body, some work voluntarily and some involuntarily. They are self-healing and grow stronger when used more often. We have three different types of muscles in our bodies. The muscles you can feel and see, and can build up by working out are called skeletal muscles. They are attached to the skeleton and come in pairs. You can move these muscles voluntarily. The muscles in your digestive system, uterus, blood vessels, arteries, esophagus and bladder are called smooth muscles and move involuntarily. Cardiac muscles are found - you guessed it! - in your heart... and fortunately move involuntarily.

All the muscles in your body crave nutrient rich food because they work by converting energy into movement. Without the right nutrients, your muscles will become weak and flaccid. In the case of skeletal muscles, they will cease to be able to fully support the body. In the case of cardiac muscles, you may experience arrhythmia (irregular heartbeats) and in the case of the smooth muscles, you may experience constipation or diarrhea, among other conditions. To keep your muscles strong and flexible, a diet rich in healthy proteins from meat or vegetables, grains and legumes is essential. The complex (healthy) carbohydrates found in whole grains, fruits and vegetables provide the necessary fuel to keep your muscles moving, and healthy fats provide extra energy, and help keep the cell membranes in your muscle tissue fluid. If you are feeding your body lots of sugar and junk, you won't get the nutrients necessary to keep all your muscular systems working as they should.

Skin

We are covered by the largest organ of the body, known as skin. Our skin protects us, and helps us release toxins in the body through sweat. Skin is comprised of the epidermis, the dermis and the subcutaneous layer. The epidermis functions as the protective barrier and contains hair follicles, nerve endings and sweat glands. The dermis is sandwiched between the epidermis and the subcutaneous layer and contains blood vessels, capillaries, hair follicles, sweat glands and nerve endings. The subcutaneous layer is the inside layer and contains blood vessels, which branch into the dermis and feed the capillaries.

Most of us have had very obvious evidence that the food we eat affects our skin. How many times have you blamed the appearance of a pimple or acne on what you ate? And what you ate was greasy, fried or full of sugar. How often have you noticed swelling or water retention due to eating too much salt? Have you ever adopted a diet purported to give you beautiful, glowing skin? Did this diet consist of foods high in anti-oxidents and healthy fats? Did you eat blueberries and salmon for a week and notice that your skin did indeed look better? Your observations are correct! If your skin looks supple, well moisturized, glowing, clear and bright, you are eating foods it likes, most likely whole foods including lots of fruits, veggies, whole grains and healthy fats. If your skin looks dull, dry, tired, grey and puffy, and you have break-outs, you are most likely eating too much processed food of one kind or another.

In this instance, you have visible proof that what you eat affects the health, and appearance of your body. Your skin is a direct reflection on the outside of what you're doing to your body on the inside. You may not be able to see the effects of junk food on your heart or liver right away, but your skin will show you almost immediately how what you're eating is impacting your body and your health. Take heed and pay attention to your skin. It will tell you long before symptoms of liver or kidney damage show up, whether or not you are feeding your body nutritionally beneficial food.

METABOLIC SYNDROME:

Metabolic syndrome (also known as Syndrome X or Insulin Resistance) is a compilation of five specific disease states. If and when they come together in one person,(hopefully they never will), they can result in a syndrome that is known to increase the risk of heart disease, stroke, coronary artery disease and diabetes. Just having three of the five indicators of metabolic syndrome, SIGNIIFCANTLY raises your risk for serious health problems. The five culprits are:

- Waist circumference greater than 35" in women and 40" in men
- Triglycerides more than 150 milligrams/deciliter
- HDLs (good cholesterol) less than 40 milligrams/ deciliter in men and less than 50 milligrams/deciliter in women
- Blood Pressure more than 130 /85 (the top number - 130 - is known as systolic, the
- bottom number - 85 - is the diastolic)
- A FASTING blood sugar of more than 100 milligrams/ deciliter

Insulin is a hormone produced in the pancreas. Certain foods, when broken down by the body, become sugar (glucose). Insulin is responsible for allowing the sugar in your blood stream to get into the cells of your body. This is their fuel and they need it to function. In cases of insulin resistance (IR) your cells lose the ability to respond to the effects of insulin, so the sugar stays in the blood. The cells do not receive the fuel they need to function properly, and as a result, you do not receive the energy you need, which will most likely cause you to feel weak, lethargic, nauseated, dizzy, lightheaded and /or sweaty. Your vision may become blurred, your heart may begin to race. Eventually, when your brain does not get the "fuel" it needs to function, it will shut down, which can result in coma. If the sugar levels in the blood are extremely high (hyperglycemia) for extended periods of time, tissue and organ damage will occur, which will lead to kidney failure and dialysis, or nerve damage in the eyes (blindness), and numbness in the legs and feet (neuropathy). Another name for all this drama is DIABETES.

CHRONIC INFLAMMATION:

Chronic inflammation of organs and tissues (internal) is not the same as inflammation of a tendon (tendonitis) or a joint bursa (bursitis). Tendinitis and bursitis can be treated with anti-inflammatory medications such as aspirin, Advil or Aleve. Chronic inflammation of the organs and tissues is the evidence of the damage that has been done to your organs and tissues over time due to the foods you're eating. Eating processed foods and refined sugars will lead to this type of inflammation and will predispose you to MANY chronic disease including cancer, atherosclerosis, rheumatoid arthritis, dementia and insulin resistance. The inflammation cannot be treated with medication (like anti-inflammatories) and is only resolved by drastic changes in diet and lifestyle.

When you are carrying excess fat, an auto-immune process is activated. Your immune cells attack your fat cells which then excrete a substance that causes inflammation in the blood vessels and organs, which is what ultimately leads to the diseases listed above. The more fatty tissue you have, the more extreme the auto-immune response can be. So the inflammation is INDIRECTLY related to the foods you eat, but is DIRECTLY related to inflammatory substances. An increase in waist circumference correlates directly with an increase of systemic chronic inflammation (see above).

The most effective treatments for chronic inflammation and insulin resistance are: weight loss, exercise, decreasing or quitting smoking and of course, revising your diet. The best foods for reversing insulin resistance and chronic inflammation are whole foods! Eat colorful, fresh fruits and vegetables; foods high in fiber, like whole grains and beans; foods high in omega-3 fatty acids, like extra virgin olive oil, avocados, salmon, tuna, nuts and seeds... all of the foods I've been advocating throughout this chapter. Stay away from all processed foods, but especially refined sugars and flours.

ADULT ONSET DIABETES:

In years past, diabetes was described as either type 1-childhood-onset or type 2-adult-onset. Due to the new phenomenon of "adult" onset diabetes showing up in children, the names have been changed (without protecting the innocent). Type 1 diabetes is caused by the inability of the pancreas to produce insulin. Unfortunately, some children are born with this deficiency. As mentioned before, insulin is the hormone needed to take glucose (sugar) out of the blood stream and put it into the cells. However, if insulin is not produced, the sugar you ingest just floats around in the blood stream instead of nourishing the cells. When the cells do not receive enough glucose, they are depleted of the energy they need to function properly. Additionally, the excess sugar in the blood will eventually damage the blood vessels. This is not a problem that can be fixed with weight loss or exercise, it can only be managed. Even though these kids must watch what they eat and stay healthy, they will need insulin from an outside source for the rest of their lives.

Type 2 diabetes is most often related to obesity and the inability of the body to USE the insulin that it produces (known as insulin resistance). This usually starts after the ages of twenty-five to thirty. Although there are two forms of type 2 diabetes (obese and non-obese), the form related to obesity is the most common. Our youth have become more sedentary as technology has expanded. That coupled with a loss of gym classes and sports in schools makes them much more inactive than any previous generation. Add that to busy parents working long hours which often forces them to turn to "quick fixes" or fast food (processed foods), and you end up with a lot of unhealthy kids.

Not only are more and more kids obese, but more often than not, as a result of over eating heavily processed foods, their weight is concentrated in their abdomen. This concentration of fat correlates very strongly with a higher incidence of insulin resistance, and ultimately diabetes. So now we have a generation of adolescents being diagnosed with a medical condition that should be "reserved" for their parents and grandparents! This is the point where many of these kids begin the journey down that long, dark road of "yo-yo" dieting and weight management "issues." These issues often stay with them for years, and are coupled with the side effects that come from long term use of medications needed to control blood sugar and prevent the disease from adversely affecting other organs.

The damage that diabetes does to the body is not pretty and gets worse as the disease progresses. If you have type 2 diabetes, and you are not willing to change your life-style or diet, even with medication, you can expect to experience deterioration of the body. Specifically, kidney damage that may lead to kidney failure and the need for dialysis, vision problems that may eventually lead to blindness, heart disease, and nerve damage to your extremities leading to the loss of fingers and toes.

So is it just me, or does anybody else think there must be a better way? There is a better way and it begins with your diet! A change in diet will have an immediate positive impact on your health. And if combined with weight loss and exercise, all together they can potentially reverse the sequela of insulin resistance. I recommend the same diet for diabetics that I do for those dealing with chronic inflammation and metabolic syndrome: clean, colorful, fresh fruits and vegetables, lean protein, complex carbohydrates and healthy fats. Stay away processed, packaged and fast foods - in other words, stay away from refined sugars and grains, trans fats and alcohol.

Being healthy is more about feeling good, than looking good. Although looking good is influenced by what you eat, many other factors contribute as well. For example, exercise, lifestyle and genetics are at the top of the list. But if you eat junk all the time, the "looking good" never happens. It's about being all you can be, and living your best life! Using the right "fuel" for your body allows you to do that on a daily basis. What's better than having good energy, sleeping well, being able to think more clearly, being alert to learn and share your gifts with your friends, family, community and the world?

Chapter Three

HOW PRIMARY FOODS AFFECT WHAT YOU EAT

What and why we eat is a much more complicated subject than you may think. Contrary to popular belief, it's not always: I'm hungry, that looks good, eat everything in sight. Humans are very complex beings. Our emotions and our personal and professional lives affect everything we do on a daily basis, 24/7. If you figure out how to put the rest of your life in balance, your eating will fall in line. Secondary Foods (veggies, fruits, carbs and proteins) feed your body, while Primary "Foods" (love, nurturing, sense of purpose, financial security, energy, health, sense of well-being) feed your heart and soul.

The concept of Primary and Secondary Foods was coined by a man named Joshua Rosenthal, the CEO and founder of the Institute for Integrative Nutrition (IIN) in New York. He believes in balance in all sectors of life. And if one area is out of whack it affects all others, including what we eat and why. He has observed that we often use Secondary Foods to comfort ourselves in times of trouble or stress. We rationalize eating when we're not actually hungry for <u>food</u>, by saying to ourselves: "I've been good, I deserve a treat," or "I need cheering up, I'm having an ice cream cone." In these instances, the truth is that we are actually in need of loving, nurturing, security, energy, hope, joy, purpose or satisfaction.

Many of the most common, yet most debilitating diseases people suffer from are due to the abuse and misuse of Secondary Foods (in the form of junk food). When we try to substitute Secondary for Primary Foods, we avoid dealing with the issues that are really troubling us and create health problems that only add to and complicate the real issues.

In this chapter I will discuss six of the Primary Foods: 1) Relationships, 2) Career, 3) Finances, 4) Physical Activity, 5) Health, and 6) Spirituality.

Relationships

If you're over thirty years old, chances are you've had your share of relationships. Some good, some... not so much. The key to supporting yourself is to make sure your relationships support you and your needs. What do you want from your relationships; what DON'T you want? This applies to casual friendships, family relationships and intimate relationships. Generally speaking, if you don't feel encouraged, accepted, supported and loved in your relationships, you are probably feeling drained, defeated and tense. Feeling drained and tense leads to feelings of resentment and anger. Experiencing emotional tension and upheaval on a daily basis can drag you down. To make ourselves feel better, we often turn to Secondary Foods (junk food). I mean really, who among us has not felt better (temporarily) after a pint of ice cream or bag of chips? But after the high comes the crash, and we're still in a bad, unsupportive and unhealthy (on multiple levels) place.

So if you're in a relationship that's not giving you what you want or need, make some changes. I know this is often easier said than done, but you must seriously consider the consequences to your overall health and well-being if you don't have the courage to make a change. Not only are you likely to suffer from the psychological stress an unsupportive relationship can create, (feelings of unworthiness, low self-esteem, lack of confidence, depression, etc...), but in an attempt to comfort yourself with junk food, you damage yourself. You damage your body and your precious health; you can shorten your lifespan or make the life you have left all about managing the diseases you've manifested by not dealing with your core issues – your relationships!

If you need help making changes in your relationships, there are plenty of resources online and in your community to guide you. Find a therapist, counselor or minister who can help you. Seek support from the healthy relationships in your life. While you're going through the process of repairing or leaving your unhealthy relationships, support yourself by meditating, working out, pampering yourself, being around people who love you, investing in meaningful work or projects. Do anything but over-indulging in Secondary Foods, which will just undermine your attempts to change by repeating those negative patterns and behaviors. Remember, relationships are a Primary Food Group and are ultimately meant to make you feel healthy and happy.

Career

Many of us spend more than 50% of our day at work. So how crazy is it to do something you don't enjoy? Now I'm not advocating that you quit tomorrow, regardless of how you feel about your job, boss or co-workers. But if the stress and/or frustration you feel in your job is pushing you into an unhealthy life style, something has to change. If you come home and your pet bird mocks you: "Not another day," clearly there is a problem. Chances are, the frustration you feel will compel you to attempt to eat your way out of your misery. That translates into eating foods that don't help you create balance in your life or support your goals. "If you always do what you've always done, then you'll always get, what you've always got." (Source unknown)

So I have to ask, "Is that you?" If it is, how much longer are you going to live like that? Always feeling out of sorts, not able to get on the right track, living a very unproductive life. Feeling adrift, out of place, unappreciated and/or off purpose, can bring up feelings of self-recrimination and self-doubt. Anger turned inward causes depression and depression can lead to a desire for sugar, and lots of it! There's nothing like sugar (especially mixed with caffeine) to create a false sense of purpose... and then a crashing sense of "why bother." It's a vicious cycle that will very quickly degrade your ability to make the changes you must make in order to discover your true purpose in life.

So now's the time to put down the Venti Double Caramel Frappuccino with extra whip and develop an action plan. Make a list, take a test, do some research, go back to school or volunteer. Anything to find your calling, your passion, your "true north." Once you find it, no matter how much of a surprise it is, don't fight it. Move towards it, no matter how long it takes. You may not be destined to change the world, but when you start living to fulfill your purpose, you just might!

Finances

We can't have a discussion about work-life balance and how it affects us without talking about finances. Money may or may not be the "root of all evil," but it definitely can be the root of MAJOR stress and anxiety. And we all know that stress and anxiety can lead to impulsive decisions, especially when it comes to food. You will likely find yourself eating when you aren't hungry and you'll make choices that will probably not be good for you. Not to mention that you'll be literally "throwing good money after bad."

In fact, if you're spending (at least) $5-$10 a day on treats from Starbucks to temporarily assuage your anxiety and stress, it can really start to add up! You could be saving that money to use on things that really matter to you, like starting a business or taking a healthy cooking class. What do you really want? What will honestly make you happy? How can you advance your future? By sucking down a Venti White Chocolate Mocha Frappuccino with extra whipped cream (550 calories), or by being your own boss and finally doing what you know you were meant to do? In the end, eating junk food as compensation for a job you don't like or due to financial stress will make you feel worse. Even demoralized and defeated. Feelings that in no way support personal progress, inspire creativity, or encourage you to make changes.

We all have to decide for ourselves how much money we require to meet our needs. Notice I did not say "to be happy," because we all know how that singular focus will end. Many people tend to ignore their calling or their purpose because the money is not "right." This can lead to so much unhappiness and discontent, not to mention wasted talent and wasted lives.

Some time ago I saw an episode of "Oprah's Lifeclass" and the topic was finding and living your truth. A caller came on and talked about how she really wanted to go into real estate and about how it was something that excited her when she thought about it as a career. But she had a very good paying job and was having trouble letting that go. She openly admitted to not liking her job, but couldn't step away from the money. Does this sound like you? Do you have one foot out the door, and the other stuck in a rut? Life is too short to straddle the fence for 30, 40, 50 years.

Start today, make an "escape plan." Give yourself a reasonable time frame to implement it. Then take the leap!! When you do what you love, it shows. People will be drawn to your positive energy. The work will come, the balance will come, and the money will come!

Physical Activity

The more you move the better you feel. The brain and the body both work better when you're in good physical shape. Most major diseases can be avoided or at least significantly curtailed with consistent exercise. We are all familiar with the cycle: the more you do, the better you feel - the better you feel the better you eat - the better you eat the more you do. Who wants to do all that exercise then put the weight back on by eating junk? It's too hard, it's too painful, it takes too much time out of your life to do that. Seriously, right now, raise your hand if you believe this is true. That's what I thought. So let's get off the merry-go-round.

A sedentary life style will slowly sap your strength and energy. You'll begin to feel more lethargic, then you'll notice how comfortable your sweat pants are, and how the imprint on the couch cushion fits... you!! You then start to crave Secondary Foods that you think will make you feel better, not physically but emotionally. And now you're on another type of merry-go-round: feel bad - eat bad - feel bad... It's one big pity party and you're the guest of honor! Stop making excuses, stop criticizing yourself, stop killing yourself (literally)! If not now, when?

So whatever you like to do, just DO IT. Walk, run, amble, swim, bike, do yoga, Pilates or Zumba. Just do something to get yourself moving. If you ask, your body will tell you what it wants and needs. What makes it feel better and what does not. Just stop, take a deep breath, and LISTEN.

Health

Obviously this book is about nutrition and making the necessary changes YOU need. Part of being healthy is dependent on the foods you eat. Not everyone should be a vegetarian, however, not everyone should eat meat and potatoes either. That's why finding what works for you is so important. What foods make you feel great? And I don't mean that temporary high you get from sugar, salt or fats. I mean what gives you energy and endurance and the feeling that you can conquer the world? Once you figure that out, you will be on the path to a happier, more fulfilled life. You will be one step closer to balance, which affects all aspects of your life.

With all the bad foods out there and the bad information about the bad foods (making them sound good), this journey is not an easy one. It must be approached one day at a time. One meal at a time. One bite at a time. This way you be begin to establish new and improved habits. Pay attention to how your food looks, smells and tastes with each bite. This routine will allow you to be more cognizant of what you are eating, and will hopefully help you make better choices.

When you are healthy, you feel good and you have energy. You are at a normal weight for your height and probably like the way you look, which gives you more confidence. When you are healthy, you maintain higher energy levels as you age and you retain the cognitive ability to continue learning and even to continue innovating. You have the emotional stability to form and keep friendships and intimate relationships. You have the stamina and courage to make changes when necessary or desired. Being "healthy" should be your goal, because your health affects ALL other aspects of your life. Optimum health requires a life-long commitment to both diet and exercise. I'm encouraging you to take your diet seriously, because what you eat has a profound effect on your over-all health. You are what you do with what you eat!

Spirituality

Spiritual nutrition feeds different people in different ways. Some people have felt a connection with God all their lives, while others are just taking the first steps on the journey. Many people follow an organized religion, its tenants and laws, while others practice being one with the universe or a higher power. There are those who do not believe in a higher power, but get sustenance out of being in nature or nurturing others.

My spirituality (Christianity) has nourished me for many years. It has given me a grounding and stability I have not found anywhere else. My beliefs have instilled in me a sense of service. They have caused me to take to heart the phrase: "There but for the grace of God, go I." Realizing that we are all connected, and being of service to others is what I feel my life must be about. Becoming a physician was a natural part of that path. Learning about nutrition and wellness, wanting to help others be their best is an extension of that.

Without a way to feel peace in your heart and love for yourself, the inclination to find solace and comfort in food can be overwhelming. Have you ever eaten when you felt lonely or hopeless or scared? We all do it and it doesn't help in the long run, does it? The only way to alleviate the fear and aloneness we have all felt at some point in our lives is to make peace with yourself and find a connection to something meaningful. Finding a community of like-minded souls can also be profoundly supportive and uplifting.

Whatever practice you chose, make it the best one for you. Make sure you feel comfortable, secure and loved. It should bring you a sense of peace when you're worried, strength when you're weak, joy when you are sad and comfort when you feel alone. Humans were not placed on earth to be isolated from one another, so make sure you're not. Feeding your body and your spirit will bring more rewards than money can ever buy.

Chapter Four

Yes, There Is Another Way And It's Not A Diet!

Making Changes

So you've decided to take the plunge. You're going to make some changes in the way you eat and the way you live. Congratulations!! There's no time like the present to get started on the first day of the rest of your life. Ok, enough of the clichés. Your first step is to clean out the kitchen pantry and the refrigerator. It is much easier to start making small changes when the temptations are removed. There is no need to empty the entire refrigerator or waste lots of money by throwing good food away, but if you are really serious about starting something new, sacrifices will have to be made.

If you have a family, they also need to be on board with your decision. These changes will affect everyone. Making the choice to change, but having your family insist all the bad foods stay "for them" will defeat you out of the gate. Below I've listed food substitutions you can make right away without causing an uproar in the family.

Substituting This for That

This is as simple as it looks! Throw out or replace the items in the OUT column with the items in the IN column.

OUT	ITEM	IN
Vegetable	Oil	Olive, Canola, Safflower
Soft	Cheese	Hard
White	Rice	Any Other Color
White	Potatoes	Sweet
Milk	Chocolate	Dark
Instant	Oatmeal	Steel Cut
Potato chips	Snacks	Unbuttered Popcorn
White	Sugar	Agave, Stevia, Raw Honey, Maple Syrup
Cow's milk	Calcium	Sesame Seeds, Collards, Kale, Almonds

Almost everything in the IN column can be found in a regular grocery store. If you have a specialty health food store in your neighborhood, I recommend making a trip there. I also recommend checking out your local farmers market for fresh, organic fruits and vegetables as well as specialty items such as cheese, dark chocolate and free-range eggs and meats. Neighborhoods in many cities around the country are now hosting farmers markets. Often you will find that much of the food at farmers markets is fresher and more affordable than you thought. Many cities also have locally run cooperative food markets, which offer local produce and meat as well as bulk foods items such as whole grains, nuts and dried fruits.

<u>Overcoming Obstacles</u>

Our next hurdle is to work on those CRAZY excuses that may hold you back. Sometimes they prevent you from getting started, sometimes they can stop you mid-stride. There will always be naysayers whenever you try to better yourself or change the status quo. There will always be "friends" who will get in your head and attempt to reinforce all the reasons you should not make changes. They have probably tried and failed or worse, have been afraid to ever try.

There are lots of ways that doubt and sabotage can seep in now that you've taken the first step. Here are some common misconceptions I've heard from clients in the past:

- I can't lose weight at my age
- Nutritious foods are too expensive
- I don't have time to prepare all that food
- I'll get too hungry if I change what I eat
- I won't lose weight eating 4-6 times a day
- It's hard to eat healthy when I go out to restaurants
- It will be really hard to change my old habits

Developing a System

Now you need to be sure that you're ready. So look in the mirror, take a deep breath and say: "Today is the first day of the rest of my life." Another cliché, but a powerful and meaningful one. Next step, pick a start date. This will help you show the world and yourself, that the time has come. This also makes you accountable and makes your decision real. Once conviction sets in, consistency will follow. That will be key to reaching your goal:

- Identify your goals (be honest with yourself)
- Set a specific start time (date and time)
- Set a specific time to meet your goal (make it realistic)
- Evaluate your Primary Foods (see Chapter Three)
- Arrange your kitchen (start clean by getting rid of as much junk food as you can without having a meltdown)
- Get your family on board (their support will be helpful, especially on the bad days)
- Choose ONE person outside of your family to tell (it increases your commitment level)
- Eat with awareness (pay attention to everything you put in your mouth)

Fact or Fiction

There is a lot of misinformation out here about health, diets, what to eat and what not to eat. Unfortunately, most of that comes from the experts, all with differing views on what works and what doesn't. However, the public also perpetuates some myths on its own. These can cause confusion and self-doubt, and can even sabotage our efforts BEFORE we get started. Take a look below and see if any of these sound familiar:

- **At my age, nobody loses weight – FICTION**
  Anybody can lose weight. The rate at which that happens and the effort it takes does change. Due to factors like loss of muscle mass with age (muscle burns more calories than fat), changes in hormone production and a more sedentary life style, weight does come off more slowly, but it DOES come off!

- **"Healthy food" is just too expensive – FICTION**
  You don't have to buy all organic to get nutritious foods. There are some foods that are safer if organic (see the Clean Fifteen listed in Chapter Five). But in the long run, fresh or frozen really is less expensive than processed, boxed or bagged. This is especially true if you factor in the probability that you'll spend less money in the long term on doctors and prescription drugs if you adopt a healthy diet.

- **I don't have time to cook every night – FACT (maybe)**
  Ok, so let's go with Plan B. Cook meals on the weekends and freeze them. During the week, just pull them out and microwave or heat. Makes it easier for your kids too.

- **I gained weight because I quit smoking – FICTION**
  You gained weight because you satisfied your oral fixation with candy, cookies and sweets. Yes, most people need something in their hands or mouth to replace the cigarette but it's all about choice.

- **If I cut back my calories, I'll be hungry all day – FICTION**

  Portion control is the cornerstone of weight loss and getting healthy. But you NEVER have to feel hungry just because you change what you eat. There are plenty of low-calorie foods that taste great, fill you up, and are good for you. And they make you feel good and give you energy.

- **Eating 4-5 times a day will only make me gain more weight – FICTION**

  How many times have you tried to lose weight by eating one meal a day? Has that ever worked? I'm guessing no. Your body and your brain need fuel 24 hours/day. The better quality the fuel, the better all your systems function. Eating three regular meals (portion control my friend) and two-three small snacks is the way to keep your fuel tank full.

- **Everyone in my family is big, it's in our genes – FICTION**

  Many physical traits and even some diseases have a genetic component. The foods you eat and the way you eat are more cultural than genetic. Learning to love family favorites is fine, but you may need to cook them differently and eat smaller portions.

- **I exercise so I can eat what I want – FICTION**

  I've heard so many overweight, out of shape people say this. And my response is always the same - in the words of Dr. Phil McGraw: "How's that workin' for ya?" Nothing could be further from the truth. You can only lose weight when calories in are LESS THAN calories out.

The Eating Plan

The Eating Plan Is Simple and Easy to Follow:

1. Set realistic goals for yourself.
2. Keep track of what you eat throughout this process and make note of how different foods make you feel, both physically and emotionally.
3. Substitute food that you know is unhealthy with healthier choices.
4. Generally speaking, all processed, pre-packaged and fast foods are unhealthy.
5. Whole foods (unrefined, unprocessed food), particularly organic, locally raised and grown foods are healthy.
6. Pay attention to what you're eating. Chew you food. Eat mindfully.
7. Start slowly and progress gradually. Be patient with yourself.

Now the real work begins! With the stresses of modern life, eating responsibly is more important than ever. Have you ever slowed down long enough to notice how you feel after you eat? Some foods make you euphoric, some energetic, some slow and bloated and some even make you feel depressed. Food affects all your body functions, so naturally your body will tell you what it likes and doesn't like by how your feel after you eat. Just because you like something (you in this case is your taste buds) does not mean it agrees with you. For example, I loved (still love) ice cream and pizza. They used to be part of my favorite lunch. Then my body started rejecting them. Translation: every time I ate dairy I experienced bloating, nausea and even diarrhea. I tried every way possible to get around this, to no avail. The thought of giving up two of my favorite foods was heartbreaking. But at 23 years old, my body said, "I've had enough!!" I could have forced the issue and continued getting sick for a few seconds of taste, or make a change.

Paying attention to your "inner food voice" is the first step to making changes in your eating plan. **Keep a food diary for one week before you start making changes (and continue keeping your food diary for as long as you are making changes to your diet).** Include exactly what you eat (even gum) and how it makes you feel. Nauseated, bloated, overly full, sleepy, hyper, unfocused, weak or happy, euphoric, satisfied, calm, energized? At the end of your first week of keeping the food diary, take a look and ask yourself where it would be easiest for you to make a change in your eating: breakfast, lunch or dinner.

If it's lunch, start with lunch. For a week, instead of having a cheese burger and large fries every day, order a burger without cheese, get a small fries instead of a large and add a salad. **Try to eat the whole salad first.** When you eat something with fiber and roughage at the beginning of your meal, it will fill you up faster and you won't be as hungry. So it will keep you from eating (and wanting) as many fries. At the end of that first week of making changes, try to eliminate the fries altogether, but keep the burger and salad.

If you're consistently eating at a fast food restaurant like McDonald's and budget is a concern, write down what you spend on lunch every day for a week and then look at what you could do with that money at home. **Making a sandwich at home is healthier and probably cheaper.** Some people say I don't have the time. I say, try preparing your food the night before. You do that for your kids don't you? What you're making at home is likely to be less expensive than eating out at fast food places every day. And chances are it's healthier (as long as you're not making bologna sandwiches with gobs of mayonnaise). Try buying freshly sliced meat from the deli, or a cooked whole chicken or turkey breast and slice it up. Use a whole grain bread, add lettuce, tomato and avocado with mustard and a smear of mayo. You get the picture...

In general (unless you do heavy physical work) eat something light, something that will keep you alert and focused, not something heavy and starchy. Have protein and vegetables and some fruit – that would be a good lunch. You don't have to have a salad, you can eat a piece of chicken or beef with broccoli or asparagus, so you have complex carbs that will keep you full and protein which will satiate you. You don't want to eat simple carbs that break down quickly, you want to eat complex carbs that break down slowly in your system so you won't get that 3pm crash and wind up hunting for coffee or sweets.

This strategy goes for anything you're eating that you <u>know</u> is not ideal, like pizza, mac & cheese, or any other creamy, cheesy pasta, a burrito with chips, fried chicken with mashed potatoes, etc... **Find a way to slowly reduce or cut out the heavy, fatty processed portion of your meals and replace it with vegetables and leaner proteins.** This is not a complex or mysterious meal plan, but one more about weaning yourself off the high calorie, heavily processed, fatty, salty, sugary foods and slowly replacing those foods with healthier choices. The point here is that it takes time to make this shift, and be aware of how you <u>feel</u>, every step of the way. As you feel better, lighter and more energetic, you will also feel encouraged to continue making the changes to your diet, until one day, you'll find yourself <u>wanting</u> a big, fresh salad with seared tuna rather than four slices of pizza.

The strategy is the same for dinner as it is for lunch, start making substitutions. If you're taking your kids to Wendy's three or four times a week, then at the very least you can order something a little more healthy from the menu – a salad instead of burger and fries... Fast food or pizza once a week is fine, but not every night and not three to four times a week. **Invest in a crock pot – throw in meat and vegetables and when you get home eight hours later, it'll be ready.** Make things on the weekend and freeze them. Come home, throw the frozen food in the microwave and you're set. You don't have to cook from scratch after you come home from work. You can pick up a roast chicken from the grocery store, pop a package of "Steamables" (fresh, frozen veggies in a pouch), in the microwave, steam and eat. You don't have to get out pots and pans and wait for the water to boil, or spend an hour cleaning up after dinner! Slicing some roast chicken and nuking a package of "Steamables" will take all of ten minutes. **Go ahead and buy food that's convenient and pre-cooked, flash-frozen veggies; frozen, pre-cooked whole grains and pre-cooked, organic meats.** Fresh is always best, but frozen (and even canned) veggies are better than mac & cheese.

If you absolutely have to have dessert after dinner, I have only one thing to say to you: portion control. **USE A**

SMALLER BOWL! Smaller dishes mean smaller servings. Psychologically, you still have a whole bowl, but you're eating less. Instead of eating ice cream with hot fudge, try coconut milk or soy ice cream with a couple of nuts for fiber and protein instead. Just try it, you may start to like it! Cut out the whipped cream, put fruit on your ice cream and cut the chocolate sauce in half. Eat half a piece of cake instead of the whole piece. Have one cookie instead of two. And try a big cup of mint or chamomile tea after dinner, BEFORE dessert, which will help cut down your desire for sugar. The liquid will fill you up and help with digestion.

If you're craving a snack before bed, I'd ask you why? If you had big dessert and are crashing and feeling hungry, you need something with fiber and protein so you don't wake up in the middle of the night feeling like you're starving. Eat a handful of nuts and a couple slices of apple.

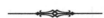

Is *breakfast* really your most important meal?? The answer is yes! Overnight your body uses all the glucose (sugar/energy) it has stored, so in the morning, it's running on empty. No matter how busy you are or what you have to do, there should always be time for a little something. Don't eat fast food, make your own "McMuffin" the night before, then just heat in microwave for a minute. (Use a whole grain muffin for more fiber.) Make a large bowl of steel cut oatmeal at the beginning of the work week and divide up into little baggies, then pop one in the microwave on the way out the door. Add cinnamon (instead of sugar) and any fruit that is handy. Eat a piece of whole grain toast with almond butter or natural peanut butter. Add a banana or some apple slices, and you're on your way. Mix your own trail mix with two-three kinds of nuts, raisins or cranberries. Maybe try oats or granola. Leave out the chocolate chips and sugar coated dried fruit. Or you can make a great protein shake with foods like bananas, apples, spinach, kale, blueberries, flax seeds, chia seeds and protein powder. All you need is a good blender and a couple of minutes! And whether you add kale or spinach or carrots, you'll only taste the fruit – I promise. These are very easy, quick "grab and go" ideas. Your body and brain will appreciate the boost!!

If you're eating three donuts and a diet coke for breakfast, okay, I get that you need your caffeine and sugar. Instead, try two donuts and a hard boiled or scrambled egg. You need some protein and you want to slowly try to cut back on the sugar. Maybe down the road, you switch from the two donuts to a bran muffin or a reduced sugar muffin and a banana. Maybe a cup of coffee with cream and a couple of teaspoons of sugar instead of a soda. **Diet soda is not better for you; artificial sweeteners can actually cause you to gain weight faster than sugar.** Sorry if you love soda, I have to be honest with you: it has ZERO nutritional value and is harming your health.

If you're the kind of person who doesn't eat breakfast and your goal is to lose weight, you'll never do it. In fact, if you skip meals in an effort to lose weight, your body's not going to burn calories very quickly. Your body is designed for survival and will do whatever is necessary to preserve itself. If your body thinks it's not going to get anything else to eat it will act as if it is starving and will only burn the minimal amount of calories it takes to function. When you do finally eat, chances are that you'll eat too much because you're hungry, and at that point your body is not going to let you break down and burn your food. Your body will hold onto it, and store what you ate as fat to ensure that it has enough energy to survive. If you don't eat, your brain doesn't have any sugar to run on, so you're going to be tired and sluggish. Then you're going to reach for a candy bar to give yourself energy. The person who eats every four hours will burn off calories quickly and efficiently because the body becomes conditioned to know it will get fuel again soon.

This brings me to the subject of snacks. **Snacking (1-2 times a day) can help keep your metabolism pumped up, if you eat the right stuff.** Start packing apples, carrots, cheese, yogurt, nuts, even popcorn and snack your way to weight loss and good health. How about dark chocolate covered blueberries, or goji berries? Fruit and fiber with dark chocolate, a win-win. Have a couple of pieces. Chew nice and slowly. That will help cut your sugar craving, and keep you from overdoing it. Snacking throughout the day really is a good thing. It's important to eat every 3-4 hours in order to keep your metabolism revved up. But that does not mean eating a full meal. The key is to curb your appetite with high fiber foods that give you energy. So here are some snacking tips to keep you feeling good and keep you going ALL day.

Snacks should be no more than 200 calories. Don't wait more than five hours between meals and snacks. It slows your metabolism and it will cause you to eat more during meals. Don't get hooked on those 100 calorie bags. You won't feel full, and you'll eat 2-3 bags. If you're craving something really sweet try something new, like dates. They have a low glycemic index (GI) so they won't raise your blood sugar like sugary snacks and desserts will. Dates are a great source of fiber, as well as polyphenols, which are important anti-oxidants (dates are even higher in polyphenols than blueberries or plums). And post workout, they provide potassium and decrease lactic acid build up in the muscle which causes soreness. So have a few dates a day, and you can go longer and harder on your next workout, while helping your overall health. If you aren't into dates, chew sugarless gum if you're craving something sweet. The artificial sugar's not great, but if it prevents you from eating something worse, I'm all for it. Remember, perfect is the enemy of good. Do your best and be conscious of your choices.

Having a party or game day should not be stressful when it comes to what you're going to eat. Most hosts will have the "standard" foods: chips/dip, nuts, pizza and of course... WINGS! There are ways to maneuver around these, and still enjoy yourself. Bring your own veggie chips (cooked in canola or olive oil), or Baked Sun Chips (multigrain are good). Eat the raw veggies with tomato salsa or guacamole (good fat) instead of creamy dip or sour cream. Eat fresh fruit (usually there is a fruit plate) and bring your own nuts, or eat with yogurt.

If you're feeling like you need a cup of coffee in the afternoon, drink a glass of water first. **If you're feeling tired you might just be dehydrated.** See how that makes you feel. Instead of a Venti Caramel Frappuccino, have a Grande without whipped cream and less caramel sauce. Then move from a Grande to a Tall. Instead of a Cinnamon Dolce Latte with whole milk, get a 2% milk latte and try cinnamon or nutmeg in it, you'll have the flavor without the extra sugar. Keep a bottle of water at your desk and drink all day long. If you don't like "plain" water, add orange, lemon or lime juice, OR cucumber and mint with stevia for sweetening. Try sparkling water like San Pellegrino or Perrier.

Making healthy choices is easier when you can plan ahead. But what happens when you're unable to control the situation? It's your boss' birthday or you're on vacation with the family and everyone is enjoying cake and ice cream. What do you do?

- Close your eyes and hope it's a dream?
- Go running from the room?
- Join in?

I say join in! It's a special occasion that only comes along once a year. Don't make yourself crazy and miss out. But make sure you focus on portion control. If you find yourself in these situations on a regular basis, you'll have to make a different decision.

- Eat ice cream in a small bowl and go light on the syrup or skip it, and add fresh fruit if available.
- Eat a bowl of sorbet instead of ice cream.
- Eat fresh fruit with a sprinkle of sugar, or yogurt if you can get it.
- Eat a small piece of cake with fruit.

Always remember to drink a glass of water BEFORE you dive in.

Are you getting the picture? **This eating plan is all about substituting healthier foods for the processed**

and fast foods you've been eating. I'm not asking you to go cold turkey. I want you to succeed, so I'm asking you to find healthier foods you like and would be willing to try in place of some of the least beneficial, most fattening foods you're eating now. **Try to upgrade to healthier choices as you're cutting back on the processed and fast food.** Decrease the bad, increase the good... and then when you get to a place where you're eating mostly good, healthy food, you can begin upgrading to better quality foods – organic, grass-fed, local etc... If you eat some things that aren't organic, that's okay as long as you get some veggies and good protein, and eliminate the sugar, fat and salt. For those of you who don't want to do a COMPLETE overhaul of your diet, start by eating ONE new healthy food a week, then two, three, four - then one a day or every other day. Slow, progressive change is the best way to get on the healthy eating track without driving yourself crazy.

One of the most important keys to success is eating mindfully. Don't just shovel food in your mouth. And NEVER, EVER eat food out of a box or bag. You'll have no idea how much you've really eaten, and before you know it, the entire bag of chips will be gone, or the sleeve of cookies will only has two left out of eight or ten. Think about why you are eating and then, whatever it is you decide to eat, pay attention to how you feel after you eat it. When you stuff food into your mouth mindlessly, you have no idea what it really tastes like, or how many calories you're consuming. The next time you start to put something in your mouth, try these steps first. Eating will become a real experience, and will likely involve less calories as well.

Eating mindfully is easier and eating is more satisfying when you take these four senses into consideration while snacking:

1. Sight: Take a look at your food. Imagine the journey it took to get to you.
2. Smell: Notice the scent and try to identify all the wonderful spices and herbs. This can enhance your appetite for fresh foods.
3. Taste: Chew slowly and take note of all the different flavors in every bite. When you eat slowly, you eat less.
4. Texture: You will be aware of this soon after you take a bite. Once the taste is gone, texture will become very apparent.

Additional recommendations that will help you practice mindful eating:

1. **When eating, limit activity to... eating:** Don't talk on the phone or watch TV or drive your car.
2. **Eat in a quiet place**: It's easier to concentrate and pay attention to what you're eating without the TV or radio.
3. **Use your NON-dominant hand:** It's harder to cut food and feed yourself using the hand with less dexterity. It will slow you down and is better for your digestion.

The transition can take as long as you need. The substitutions can be made at your discretion with the understanding that your goal is to decrease and eventually eliminate the majority of processed foods from your diet:

Sample Meal Substitutions for Four Weeks
Breakfast - Week One:
2 fried eggs (fried in butter)

4 slices of bacon (pork)

2 slices of white bread toast with butter and jelly

1 large coffee with cream and 2 teaspoons of sugar

(at work) 1 large coffee with cream and 2 teaspoons of sugar

(first meal may be typical client meal)

Breakfast - Week Two:
1 large glass of water

2 scrambled eggs (fried in Organic Olive Oil Cooking Spray – PAM or any other brand)

4 slices of bacon (pork)

2 slices of wheat bread toast with peanut butter and naturally sweetened fruit spread

1 large coffee with cream and 1 teaspoon of sugar

(at work) 1 large coffee with cream and 1 teaspoon of sugar

Breakfast - Week Three:
1 large glass of water

2 hard or soft-boiled or poached eggs

2 slices of bacon (beef or turkey)

1 slice of whole or sprouted grain toast with nut butter and naturally sweetened fruit spread

1 medium coffee with cream and 1 teaspoon of sugar

(at work) 1 medium coffee with cream and 1 teaspoon of sugar

Breakfast - Week Four:

1 - 2 large glasses of water

1 - 2 hard or soft boiled or poached eggs

½ cup steel cut oatmeal with a handful of raw nuts and raw organic honey

1 small coffee with cream and 1 teaspoon of sugar (or no sugar) (at work) 1 small coffee with cream and 1 teaspoon of sugar (or no sugar)

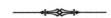

Lunch/Dinner – Week One:

2 pieces of fried chicken

1 small salad

1 large serving of Mac & Cheese

1 medium/large Pepsi

½ pint Rocky Road ice cream

Lunch/Dinner – Week Two:

2 pieces of fried chicken

1 medium salad

1 serving of stir fried veggies with ½ cup of cheese

1 small/medium sweet potato with a tablespoon of butter

1 small Pepsi

1 medium glass of water

2 scoops of ice cream

Lunch/Dinner – Week Three:

1-2 pieces of grilled chicken

1 medium salad

1 serving of steamed veggies with a teaspoon of butter, herbs or spices

1 small/medium sweet potato with a teaspoon of butter

1 large glass of water

1 -2 cups of fresh fruit or a scoop of sorbet

Lunch/Dinner – Week Four:

1 grilled chicken breast

1 medium/large salad

1 serving steamed veggies with a dash of olive oil, herbs or spices

1 small/medium baked sweet potato with a dash of olive oil, herbs or spices (no butter)

1 large glass of water

1 cup of fresh fruit

Fast food restaurants have different options that can be categorized as "bad, good, better." This is a great example of the mantra: "perfect is the enemy of good." If you eat a healthy breakfast and dinner, you can fall off a little at lunch. It would be best for you to take your lunch to work, but if that's not possible and you're stuck eating fast food, try to mitigate the damage by making the best choices you can:

Chipotle

Salad or a Bowl vs. Taco or Tortilla

Brown Rice vs. White Rice

Chicken or Tofu vs. Beef

Tomato Salsa vs. Corn Salsa

Beans - any

Veggies - any

½ to ¼ the amount of cheese or sour cream

½ the amount of guacamole (good fat)

Skip the side order of chips

Panera Bread

Steel Cut Oatmeal with Fruit or Yogurt Parfait vs. Egg/Cheese or Spinach Bacon Soufflé

Turkey/Avocado Sandwich vs. Italian Combo

Tuna Salad vs. Fontana Grilled Cheese

Mediterranean Veggie vs. Bacon Turkey Bravo

Smoked Ham/Cheese vs. Asiago Steak

Mediterranean Shrimp vs. Chicken Cobb

Caesar Salad vs. Fuji Apple Chicken

Spinach Power Salad vs. Thai Chicken

With the exception of the New England Clam Chowder, all the soups are nutritious and low calorie. By contrast, none of the pasta dishes are under 450 calories/servings and contain a fair amount of fat and salt.

McDonald's

Egg McMuffin vs. Sausage McMuffin or Chicken Biscuit

Water or Coffee vs. Milk

Fresh Fruit and Yogurt vs. Pancakes

McDouble Burger with Cheese (Grilled chicken even better) vs. Big Mac or Angus Deluxe

Small Fries vs. Large Fries

Grilled Chicken Salad vs. Caesar Salad

Unsweetened Tea, Coffee or Water vs. ANY Soda

<u>Kentucky Fried Chicken / KFC</u>
Baked Chicken vs. Fried Chicken/Extra Crispy
Corn on the Cobb (no butter) vs. Mac and Cheese
Cole Slaw vs. Buttered Biscuits
Green Beans vs. Potato Wedges
Chicken Pot Pie vs. KFC Bowl
Unsweetened Tea, Coffee or Water vs. ANY Soda

If you've read this far, I assume you're serious about making changes in your life and finally putting yourself first! If you love and appreciate your amazing body, it will give you back the energy and joy you've been missing. Give yourself the gift of good health! YOU ARE WORTH IT!

Chapter Five

STAYING ON TRACK

How does anyone manage to stay on track when trying to diet or eat healthy? This is the age old question for people trying to change their eating habits. You don't have to be perfect, just consistent. Here is a list of strategies you can employ to help you stick with your new Eating Plan:

1. **Drink more water.**

   When you are dehydrated, you can become fatigued, which can cause you to crave sugar. When you get the munchies or cravings, try drinking an 8 ounce glass of cool (not cold) water. Cool or room temperature water is more easily digestible. It will fill you up and curb the cravings so you don't reach for the junk. I recommend drinking 64 ounces of water a day, but I know that's not realistic – so if you can get four to six 8 ounce glasses of water down, you're doing great! If you don't like drinking water, try flavoring it with fresh squeezed orange, lemon or lime juice, or try a sprig of mint with sliced cucumbers for a truly refreshing drink. If you have to, I'd much prefer that you drink something like "Crystal Light" rather than soda. Splenda is not great, but better than all the calories in soda. Because dehydration manifests itself as hunger, always drink a full glass of water before you sit down to eat. It aids in digestion and will help to keep you from overeating.

2. **Increase veggies (sweet and green).**

Increasing the amount of veggies you eat will increase your fiber intake, which will make you feel full faster. Carbohydrates in vegetable form have plenty of good, unrefined sugar. If you're craving sugar, that craving will diminish if you eat vegetables (particularly sweet potatoes and carrots) because your blood sugar will go up to the point where your body will get what it needs to satisfy your desire for sugar. The great thing about veggies is that you can eat as many as you want, provided you're not adding cheese sauce or butter or too much salt. Sautéing with a little olive oil or steaming with spices or herbs is fine. If you don't like veggies solo, combine them with other foods: soups, casseroles, omelets or smoothies. One of the fastest, most convenient ways to maximize your intake of veggies is by eating them in blended smoothies (rather than juicing them) because you retain the pulp (fiber), and vitamins, minerals and enzymes, particularly if you drink it immediately after blending (before oxidation sets in). Smoothies require no measuring and minimal prep work. Just throw your favorites in a blender, press start and drink. Boost your brain power with more anti-oxidants and anthocyanins (found in red cabbage and blueberries). Fight cancer with "green drinks," made with leafy greens like kale, spinach and parsley. Need more energy, throw in some foods like beets, kale and carrots, which will increase blood flow to muscles and the brain. Adding some protein powder will slow the absorption of sugar and keep you full longer.

3. **Increase fresh fruit (especially from local providers).**

   If you eat fresh fruit instead of sugary treats, you will curb your cravings and avoid the sugar spike and crash you experience with candy, cookies, etc... Many fruits are fairly high in sugar, so you might want to eat fewer bananas, grapes and cantaloupe, and more blueberries, raspberries, apples, kiwi, oranges and grapefruits (check out the glycemic values of fruits online). However, because fruit is a complex carbohydrate, you will not have the crash you have with a candy bar even if you eat a high sugar fruit. If you want to slow down the sugar going into your system even more (which will keep you satiated for longer), eat your fruit with a little protein - nuts, nut butter, cheese, cottage cheese or plain yogurt.

4. **Decrease processed foods.**

   If you've read this far, you have a pretty good idea of how bad processed foods are for your body. If you haven't stopped eating processed foods, you must learn to read food labels (see "How to Read a Food Label" at the end of this chapter) so you are able to choose foods that are lower in sodium, sugar and trans fats. Processed foods are killing all of us little by little every day. The food industry makes them so enticing and taste so good that they are hard to resist. A good place to start weaning yourself off processed food is to step away from all sodas, canned or bottled juices, and frozen coffee concoctions. Excess and artificial sugars make you hungry faster and have no nutritional value. Add different fruits and veggies to your meals every day. This will give you more variety and let your body start developing a taste for natural sugar. Last but not least, limit yourself to ONE fried food item per week. You have to start somewhere, and in 3-4 weeks you'll miss it less and less... Don't consider it cheating. If it's controlled and built into your eating plan, then it's not cheating. Try to limit the "less healthy stuff" to the weekends, two days at first, then just one. If you plan for this, you won't feel guilty and it will give you strength to get through the rest of your week!

5. **Exercise thirty minutes every day (even if it's in ten minute increments).**
   A lot of people say they don't have time to exercise even 30 minutes a day. If you can't get up and walk around the office, try standing at your desk instead of sitting, especially when you're on the phone. Do some deep knee bends, lunges, stretches or jumping jacks. Sitting for hours on end has been proven to be detrimental to your health and take years off your life! So even if it's just for ten minutes before or after lunch, walk around your building with a friend. It's easier to stay committed

to your work out when you have someone to hold you accountable. Always take the stairs! If you work from home, get up once an hour (use a timer) and stretch or walk or do jumping jacks. Jump rope, run in place, do deep knee bends or lunges. Walk around the block a few times before or after breakfast or dinner. Take your partner or spouse and kids with you. Or you could always walk your dog (you may have to get one first, but that's okay). At the end of the day when you're watching TV, run in place, do jumping jacks or yoga stretches during commercials. There is an extensive amount of research showing that getting in at least 30 minutes of activity a day - even if it is broken up into 10 minute increments - will help to lower your blood pressure, lower your heart rate and help you lose weight (depending on what you're eating). If you exercise during the day, chances are you won't need that 3pm cup of coffee. Only thirty minutes of exercise a day can smash cravings and quell hunger. You know you're worth thirty minutes a day!

6. **Learn to cook.**
   One of the best reasons to learn to cook is so you know what's in your food. When you go to a restaurant, you have no idea what the cooks in the back are doing – regardless of what it says on the menu. You don't know what's been on the grill or what's been dropped on the floor. If you're trying to lose weight or get healthier, cooking your own food is one of the best ways to do it. Find cookbooks that show you how to prepare foods you like. Or keep it simple, sauté or steam veggies (there

are frozen veggies called "Steamables" that you can pop in the microwave) and broil a piece of fish or chicken, create a chopped vegetable salad with boiled egg on top, get a rice cooker (for all different kinds of whole grains), use a crock pot or make one meal a protein shake. Cook large amounts on the weekend, then split into small "grab and go" meals. You don't have to spend hours in the kitchen to eat delicious, healthy food!

7. **SLOW DOWN and chew your food.**

   As you break your food down by chewing, you release nutrients and initiate the digestive process. When the food hits the stomach and small intestines, the rest of the digestion process goes more smoothly. This means that the nutrients are more easily assimilated by the body, and as a result, are better utilized. Chewing at least 30-50 times, until the food in your mouth is liquefied, will relieve your digestive system from having to work so hard and will most likely prevent stomach aches and gastrointestinal issues. Most of us won't chew that long, but if you keep that number in your mind when you eat, it will slow you down.

8. **Keep affirming and updating your goals – stay true to yourself.**

   Try eating naked – just kidding! But not really. Pay attention to your body. Don't just look at yourself with clothes on. That can give you a false sense of security. But don't become obsessed with your abs, thighs or rump either. And please don't become a slave to the scale. That can derail all your hard work in one day!! Figure out what you want to change to make yourself feel better, stronger, healthier, and then go for it. If you want to lose weight stay focused on how you FEEL. Do you feel better? Are your clothes looser? What were your original goals? Did you want to be able to play with your kids for an hour in summer, or walk to the store three blocks away without collapsing? Have you reached these goals? And if the answer is yes, take the credit for the success, then set new ones.

Confronting Cravings

TO CRAVE: To desire intensely; to need urgently. That sounds about right. Especially when it comes to sugar, salt or fat. Cravings can happen any time, day or night, to anyone. Stop for a minute and write down WHEN you crave certain foods and what they are. What event or feeling or time of day do the cravings consistently coincide with? How do you feel when you first get the craving (before it's satisfied)? And more importantly, how do you feel after you eat or drink that special thing that makes the craving go away?

Have you ever stopped to think about WHY you crave the foods you do? Is it because you're stressed, or tired, or sick? Rarely, if ever, is it because you're hungry. That's just not how cravings work. Usually when you crave something it's because of the feeling the food you crave gives you and the chemicals that are produced in the brain when you eat it. It has nothing to do with willpower or being "strong" enough to resist. You can be the most disciplined person in the world, but it may not be enough. The body wants what the body wants. Not because it's greedy or wants to binge on junk food. Not because it's hungry or it needs more to eat.

Cravings are actually associated with the pleasure centers in the brain. The body responds best when it's "happy" or when it "feels good." The foods we crave most often are sugar and salt. Both of these increase the production of neurotransmitters (chemicals in the brain) that make us feel happy. For example, eating foods like cake, cookies and candy, causes an increase in dopamine and epinephrine in the body. These neurotransmitters produce a sense of well-being and happiness, and make you feel up-beat and energetic (temporarily). Salty foods, like chips, pretzels and pizza cause the neurochemical, serotonin, to be released into the brain. This also makes you feel happier and at peace (also temporarily). It is called "comfort food" for a reason. Dopamine and serotonin are used in many of the common anti-depressants that are currently on the market.

Denial of your favorite foods causes you to want them even more. That results in frustration, and more importantly obsession with that food. Then the only way to satisfy the pleasure centers is to binge on that thing you've been denying yourself. AND YOU KNOW THAT WILL END BADLY FOR YOU!

There are two hormones that play important roles in appetite and cravings - Leptin and Cortisol. Leptin is Greek for "thin" and it is associated with satiety. It is stored and secreted by adipose tissue (fat cells). It regulates hunger and tells you when to stop eating. By monitoring the energy level your body needs, it knows when your intake of energy (food calories) has met those needs. Overweight people produce excessive amounts of

Leptin. Ironically, this does not make them stop eating, rather, they become Leptin resistant. This causes the brain to ignore signals to stop eating.

Factors that may increase Leptin resistance include:

- Excessive consumption of simple carbs (sugar)
- Decreased sleep
- High stress
- Insulin resistance

Cortisol, known as the stress hormone is produced in the adrenal gland (a small gland that sits on top of the kidney). It is produced as part of the "fight or flight" response to a stressful/ dangerous situation. Chronically high levels of cortisol cause many deleterious effects on us both physically and mentally. Chronic stress and high cortisol also cause us to crave high fat, high carbohydrate foods which invariably results in overeating. (Remember when we crave, we're not usually hungry).

Here are some ways to keep your cortisol levels down:

- RELAX - whatever that means to you - meditate, exercise, listen to music, go for a walk.
- Get enough sleep.
- Learn to control your stress - you can't prevent it, but you can learn to modulate your response.

Here are a few more strategies for curbing cravings before they begin:

- Drink lots of cool, not cold, water especially at the onset of a craving.
- Eat more whole grains. You don't have to give up all carbs, but you can choose better. Brown instead of white rice, sweet instead of white potatoes, fruits and veggies instead of chips.
- Stay away from "low fat" or "diet" foods. The reason those foods are still tasty is because low fat means MORE SUGAR.
- Eat breakfast!! When you eat high fiber, filling foods, you won't crave sugary snacks throughout the day.

Ultimately, the only truly effective way to eliminate unhealthy food cravings is to gradually wean yourself off the sugar, fat and salt you've been using to "self-medicate," while simultaneously establishing and reinforcing behaviors that reduce stress and promote inner peace and happiness. Succumbing to your cravings over and over again reinforces your "need" for the food that is giving you only temporary relief from exhaustion and your feelings of depression or anxiety. It becomes a vicious cycle and will most likely lead to serious weight and health problems. By addressing the underlying life-style issues that are creating stress, anxiety, sleeplessness and/or depression in your life, you stand a much better chance of curbing and eventually eliminating cravings for junk food. For more great suggestions on "better" foods and snacks, especially when eating out, read the book, *Eat This, Not That! Thousands of Simple Food Swaps that Can Save You 10, 20, 30 Pounds -- or More!* By David Zinczenko and Matt Goulding, and get started on the right road.

How to Read a Food Label

Learning how to read a food label is crucial especially if you are eating processed, pre-packaged foods. In order to get a thorough overview of what means what on food labels, I recommend that you check out the FDA and Mayo Clinic websites. On the "Nutrition Facts" label you'll want to note how many servings are in one package, so you don't inadvertently eat the entire package. Later you may realize that it was meant to feed four people and each serving was 500 calories. In the near future the FDA will be changing the way it labels foods. The serving sizes will be what people really eat (1 cup versus ½ or ¾) so you get the full picture of how many sugar, salt and fat grams you are ingesting.

Check out the calories from fat and note whether the fats are trans, saturated or unsaturated fats. Unsaturated is generally better, through a <u>small</u> amount of saturated fat is necessary for a healthy diet. Stay away from trans fats and hydrogenated and partially hydrogenated fats! They are completely foreign to the body. It can't metabolize or use them, so it just stores them. Check out the amount of sodium and sugar in your packaged foods. You should be eating no more than 1.5 to 2.3 grams of sodium per day and no more than 25 grams for women and 35 grams for men of sugar per day. One teaspoon of sugar is 5 grams. This should give you a baseline to follow when putting sugar in coffee or on cereals. Also make note of the amount of dietary fiber listed. Is there any? The more fiber you eat, the better!

Look carefully at the ingredients list on your packaged foods. My rule of thumb is, if I can't pronounce the ingredient and I have no idea what it is, it's probably not something I should be eating! I know this is a bit simplistic, but it's not entirely without merit. Keep a look out for the most common preservatives used in packaged, processed foods. Some of them are: propionic acid, nitrates and nitrites, and benzoates (BHA, BHT). Other undesirable (unhealthy) additives to be on the watch for are: anything listed as "artificial," high fructose corn syrup (even worse for you than sugar), and monosodium glutamate (MSG). Also be alert to false advertising. For example, many cereals claim to contain "whole grains," which are good for you. Mostly this claim is not true. If you read the ingredients list carefully, you'll see that there are no or very little actual whole grains added.

Have you ever checked the labels of different foods and wondered what "low-fat" or "all natural" really means? The food industry slaps these labels on to confuse and manipulate us. So it's time to take control and find out what you're REALLY eating:

- **Low Calorie/Light** - These are NOT the same thing. Low calorie means specifically 40 or less calories per serving. "Light" refers to color flavor or texture!! So don't be fooled.
- **Multigrain** - This refers to two or more grains in the product. However, they are not necessarily WHOLE (unrefined) grains. You need to make the distinction.
- **Sugar** - REDUCED means 25% less than original product. LOW means absolutely nothing. No standard exists. NONE means no sugar was added during

preparation or cooking. And FYI - FRUCTOSE is sugar. SO IS MALTOSE, DEXTROSE AND LACTOSE.

Here are a few more tips and things to REALLY pay attention to specifically in reference to meat, dairy and poultry:

- **USDA Certified Organic** - These animals have not had any antibiotics per government inspection.
- **American Grassfed Certified** - This also certifies that the animals have not had any antibiotics. 100% grass fed is NOT the same thing. It means the animals were fed grass, but it is not guaranteed that the animals were not given antibiotics.
- **Animal Welfare Approved** - These animals have been given antibiotics, but ONLY when ill, and slaughter is delayed twice the regular period after they finish.
- **Certified Raised and Handled** - This is endorsed by ASPCA. These animals are also given antibiotics ONLY when ill and under a vet's care. This is NOT same as American Humane Certified!
- **Wild Caught Fish** - You should always eat WILD caught fish. Farm fed can be "fed" anything.
- **Natural** - THIS MEANS ABSOLUTELY NOTHING!! They can be fed anything and antibiotics are not off limits. This goes for human and pet foods.
- **Antibiotic Free** - Again, this means nothing. Don't fall for the hype.
- **Extra Lean** - According to US Food and Drug standards, extra lean means something very specific. For a 100 gram serving, less that 5 grams of total fat, less

than 2 grams of saturated fat and less that 95 milligrams of cholesterol. So this is not an arbitrary label and is one you can count on.

The best way to make sure you are eating food that is truly good for you, as I've been advocating all along, is to avoid processed, packaged, pre-prepared and fast foods completely. If this is impossible for you, learn to read labels and choose foods with lower amounts of sodium, sugar and fat. Choose foods that are labeled "Organic." Choose foods that actually contain whole foods, such as whole or sprouted grains, nuts, fruits and vegetables. Choose baked rather than fried chips, choose frozen rather than canned fruits and vegetables, choose packaged meats that are fresher (they have an expiration date) rather than heavily preserved meats (salami, Spam, bologna).

Top Foods to Buy Organic

There are many good reasons why organic foods cost more. The extra steps needed to make sure no pesticides or antibiotics are used requires time, energy and other protective measures. I know it's not always possible to buy organic and there are some fruits and vegetables that are fine to eat even if not organic (listed below), but I want you to consider the cost to your body when it has to find a way to process, digest, store and eliminate the chemicals and hormones in most non-organic food.

A lot of people want to eat organic but don't know where to start. Below is a list of what's known as the "dirty dozen." This is a list of fruits and veggies that if at all possible should be organic due to the large amount of pesticide residue:

Apples
Celery
Cherry Tomatoes
Cucumbers
Grapes
Nectarines
Peaches
Potatoes
Spinach
Strawberries
Summer Squash
Sweet and Hot Peppers

Now the good news! Here are the "Clean Fifteen." These are the foods that you don't need to buy organic unless you want to:

Asparagus
Avocado
Cabbage
Cantaloupe
Sweet Corn
Grapefruit
Kiwi
Mango
Onions
Papaya
Pineapple
Sweet Peas

Have you ever thought about the fact that organic boxed foods (like cereal) may be processed? Even though the ingredients are certified organic (wheat, rice flakes), they are still washed out via processing. The amount of fiber SHOULD be off the charts, but it's usually only 1-2 grams per serving! And the sugar content – Oh my gosh! Organic cane syrup, honey, molasses or brown sugar, is STILL SUGAR. So you can end up with 8-10 grams per serving, while the "healthy" conventional cereals have 11-12grams. So in addition to the organic certification, look for the high fiber, low sugar and LOW GLYCEMIC seal. Then just add some fresh fruit, and you'll feel great.

The ABC's of Eating Healthy

There are a lot of "everyday" foods out there that are also good for you. Despite what you might think, regular, everyday foods have all the vitamins, minerals and antioxidants you need. Supplements are nice, but not always absorbed well and not always what they seem to be. The more colorful your plate, the better off you'll be. So check these out and try to add at least ONE to your diet EVERY WEEK:

- **Sweet Potatoes** – A great source of vitamin C, potassium, beta-carotene, anti-oxidants and fiber. This sweet treat produces a hormone that turns off the hunger signal in the brain and curbs your craving for processed sugar!
- **Mangoes** – A great source of vitamins C and A. Helps lower blood pressure with high levels of potassium.

- **Greek Yogurt** – Thick, creamy and a great snack anytime. It has a whopping 18 grams of protein per serving and is best eaten plain with fresh fruit.
- **Broccoli** – A great source of vitamin C, vitamin K, folic acid and daily fiber.
- **Salmon (wild caught)** – The omega-3 fatty acids are not only great for your heart and blood pressure, but they help burn fat!
- **Garbanzo Beans** – More fiber (yay), more protein (yay), plus iron and zinc, all good for tissues and bones. Mix with meats, salads, brown rice or couscous.
- **Watermelon** – Vitamins A and C and a big dose of lycopene (a powerful antioxidant). A delicious way to hydrate and get a boost from <u>natural</u> sugar.
- **Butternut Squash** – So easy to cook - peel, dice, bake or make a soup! Full of fiber and vitamin C.
- **Spinach** – This low calorie, dark leafy green is loaded with lots of fiber and iron, and tastes great sautéed, in salads or in smoothies.
- **Soybeans (organic/non-GMO)** – This low calorie food is one of the best non-meat sources of pure protein.
- **Apples (organic)** – The high fiber content of this low-glycemic fruit will fill you up and can decrease cholesterol levels over time. The vitamin C content can also boost immunity. So try a small apple BEFORE lunch or dinner - it will curb your appetite, aid digestion and keep you healthy!
- **Brussels Sprouts** – The sulfur compounds in this vegetable can block tumor growth. Also found to

decrease inflammation caused by rheumatoid arthritis and other inflammatory diseases.

- **Basil** - Contains the compound known as eugenol which is known to block carcinogenic activity in cervical cancer.
- **Kale** - <u>The</u> super food! It has tons of vitamin K which is good for preventing heart disease and LOTS OF FIBER, FIBER, FIBER, which aids in the prevention of colon cancer.
- **Eggplant** - Its beautiful purple skin has anti-aging properties, and thanks to nasunin, it also fights cancer and slows the progression of Alzheimer's by blocking those nasty free radicals.
- **Red Bell Pepper** - One of the best sources of vitamin C - also known to increase collagen production, which helps prevent wrinkles.
- **Quinoa** – A complete non-meat protein. This seed, which is prepared and eaten like a grain, builds muscle and burns fat.
- **Tomatoes** - Filled with a powerful, life-saving antioxidant called LYCOPENE! Can help protect you from many cancers like prostate, breast and lung. Also helps lower the "bad" cholesterol, which can prevent heart attacks.

Strawberries (organic only)

These delicious, sweet berries have multiple health benefits, making them that much sweeter:

- Strawberries can lower your risk for a heart attack, especially if you're UNDER 40 years old. The redder the berry, the more anthocyanin, which is cardio protective.
- Bright red strawberries can whiten your teeth. The large amount of polyphenols, only second to coffee, help to inhibit the breakdown of sugar in the mouth, leaving less sugar residue to cause cavities.
- In addition to fiber and folate, one cup of strawberries gives you 163 % of daily vitamin C. All that for only 46 calories and great taste!
- One of the best known anti-cancer foods. Strawberries have been shown to prevent esophageal cancer, and inhibit tumor growth in some lung cancers.

So, you've got a great tasting food that helps your heart, health and smile. What more can you ask for from your food!!

Watermelon

Summer time is the BEST time to eat fresh fruit. It's everywhere, in every size, shape and color. So you don't have any excuses. If you're staying active, you need to stay hydrated. One word: WATERMELON!

FUN FACTS:
- IT REALLY IS ABOUT 92 % WATER. So have a piece when it's cold and you're hot. Great after a workout.
- VERY FEW CALORIES. An entire cup is only 46 calories. It's a good source of fiber as well.

- LYCOPENE. This is one of the strongest cancer fighting substances we have. Watermelon has MORE lycopene than tomatoes!!

So let's review: Watermelon - it taste good, it's good for you and it keeps you hydrated. Can you say that about a Popsicle?

Fall Vegetables

Just because summer has come and gone, does not mean all the good produce is gone too. There are lots of great foods still left to be eaten. Here are a few:

- **Squash** - All the beautiful types - Acorn, Butternut and Spaghetti – are all in full bloom. They are high in **carotenoids,** which is converted to vitamin A. This is good for your heart and your eyes. Squash is also high in iron and vitamin C, and both are needed more this time of year.
- **Pumpkin** - Don't just think pie! Pumpkin in soup has a sweet, creamy taste and it's also high in vitamins A and C.

Garlic

If you really want to enhance the flavor of your food, try adding some garlic. Just the smell in the kitchen makes you reach for a good glass of (red) wine in anticipation of what's to come. Garlic has many health benefits as well:

- Lowers cholesterol and can have a direct, positive effect on blood pressure. As it breaks down, it releases a substance that relaxes the blood vessel wall. This in turn lowers the pressure.
- It has been found to modulate blood sugar in diabetics.
- The sulfur compounds released in garlic as it breaks down have been known to partially inhibit growth of certain cancer cells.
- It gives your immune system a boost when taken in supplement form.

After you've enjoyed that great dish with lots of extra garlic, you can get rid of "garlic breath" by chewing on parsley or drinking milk. To get it off your hands, rub them with lemon, salt or baking soda – then rinse!

So don't shy away from this AWESOME spice. It can do so much for you, and taste good too. What more could you ask for?

Cooking Oil

We all know how good olive oil is for you, but don't forget about the other beneficial oils. Next time you're in the store, pick one of these up and give it a try:

- **Pistachio Oil** – Contains large amounts of phytosterols which reduce the risk of certain cancers. It also helps decrease the amount of cholesterol absorbed into the body.
- **Avocado Oil** - Has a very high smoke point (510 degrees vs. 325 for olive oil), which makes it safer for frying and

broiling. It's also high in MONO-saturated fats which help lower "bad "cholesterol.

- **Pumpkin Oil** - A good source of omega-3 fatty acids, and high in tocopherols which fight free radicals and slow the aging process. It also decreases systemic inflammation, which can help decrease arthritis pain.

Protein

Protein, along with fats and carbohydrates are essential for life. But just how much protein a day do you need? And how do you get it? Many say meat and dairy, others say beans and soy products. It's your choice, but you need to get your grams. It's recommended that protein be about 20% of your total daily calories. If you are over 65 years old, you may need a little more. Protein and amino acids are the building blocks for muscle, and help regulate metabolism. Protein also helps you feel full faster and longer, resulting in less intake of food. This can contribute to weight loss and better health. Without it, muscle breakdown can occur. If muscle breakdown becomes extensive, it can lead to a multitude of problems and eventually, kidney failure.

There are EIGHT essential amino acids that your body can't make, so you must ingest them. Complete proteins are animal based like meat, chicken, fish and eggs. Incomplete proteins include plant based foods like beans, rice, almonds, pumpkin seeds and soy beans. These have lower amounts of protein, but you can still get all you need with a varied diet. This formula will give you an idea of how much protein you need a day to maintain muscle mass and stay healthy: **YOUR WEIGHT x 0.4 = recommended grams of protein per day.**

For your information, the following chart from WebMD. com lists grams of protein per serving of various foods:

4 ounces roasted chicken breast without skin = 35 grams protein

4 ounces ground sirloin, broiled = 30 grams protein

4 ounces pork tenderloin, roasted = 25 grams protein

4 ounces salmon, broiled = 29 grams protein

1 cup non-fat milk = 8 grams protein

1 cup light vanilla soy milk = 6 grams protein

1 ounce reduced fat cheese = 7 grams protein

1 ounce soy cheese (mozzarella) = 6 grams protein

½ cup of beans = about 7 grams protein

½ cup fresh green soy beans = 16 grams protein

3 ounces extra firm tofu = 8 grams protein

2 egg whites (1/4 cup egg substitute) = 7 grams protein

6 ounces yogurt = 5 grams protein

1 cup broccoli = 4 grams protein

¾ cup whole grain cereal = about 6 grams protein

Eggs

Eggs are one of the best sources of pure protein. They are easy to prepare, fairly portable and good snack food. The large ones are only 60-70 calories (no carbs or fat). They are a good source of vitamin E, selenium, lutein and omega-3 fatty acids. The shell color really doesn't matter. It's up to you what type you want to buy, but if you can afford to buy "cage free," do it.

Knowing that the hen was treated humanely, and produced less stress hormones while producing the eggs, is a plus for everyone. And if you can go organic, please do! However, (and you knew this was coming), there is that cholesterol issue. As simple and clean as they are, eating four eggs every day is over-kill. If you have issues with heart disease and/or high cholesterol (get it checked if you're not sure), then eat them sparingly. You don't have to give them up, but no more than ONE a day – please!

Beans

Believe it or not, some carbs CAN help you lose weight. But you have to eat the right kind. High fiber foods like beans, release glucose (sugar) s l o w l y into the blood stream which does not cause a spike in your insulin. The sugar can be used as energy and will not be stored as fat! Also, beans are a great source of important minerals like thiamine, folate and iron. Darker beans, like kidney, contain more anti-oxidants which aid in the fight against cancer. Just 2-4 cups per week will make a difference.

Seeds

By adding seeds to your diet, you can easily increase your fiber intake while enjoying the many delicious varieties. When you sprinkle seeds into cereals, smoothies or salads, you can add as much as 12-15 grams of fiber without adding too many extra calories. Check out these seeds and see how you can use them to make one of your good dishes great!

- **Flaxseeds** - One of the most common seeds that can be added to almost anything. They have cancer prevention components and are high in omega-3 fatty acids and lignans, which make them good for fighting heart disease and stroke as well.
- **Hemp Seeds** - These seeds are considered a COMPLETE protein as they contain all the essential amino acids. They're also high in magnesium which decreases diabetes risk.
- **Buckwheat Seeds** - Lots of fiber which fills you up and aids digestion. They're also rich in PRE-biotics, so you get an immunity boost as well.
- **Wheat Germ** - The old favorite, especially for your oatmeal and protein shakes - packed with vitamins E, B and folate. This protects against colon cancer and stroke.

Immune System Boosters

Here are a few easy ways to tweak your diet to support your immune system so you never miss a single party during the holiday season!

- Switch your morning "joe" to green tea – a direct boost to your immune system.
- Engage in moderate cardio-exercise - doesn't wear your body down and causes less injury than strenuous workouts.
- For a quick energy fix, eat light fruits with a handful of nuts. Stay away from heavy carbs and sugars.

Healthier Holidays

We all get nervous around the holidays when it comes to parties. You want to enjoy yourself, but don't want to overdo it. So here are a few tricks you can use to eat, drink and be merry without the worry:

- Make sure you HYDRATE well all day, before the party. And don't let the drinking get out of hand.
- Eat a healthy snack BEFORE the party. That way you won't be starving and just shovel food in when you arrive.
- Always choose the FRESH appetizers (crudité, sushi, fruit).
- Go ahead, enjoy - have dessert, but skip the whipped cream, chocolate sauce or ice cream. That helps leave a lot of calories "on the side."
- NO means NO. When you're full, stop eating! Don't feel you must continue because the host insists.
- And finally, have a plan for exercising THE NEXT DAY. Make sure it's built into your busy schedule so you can burn off the extra calories.

Eat Your Scraps

As hard as we try every week, it seems like we're always throwing away food. Sometimes it's unavoidable, sometimes necessary and ALWAYS frustrating. But there are a few foods that produce healthy scraps. Really, it's true! They have a lot more nutrients than you think. Try these tips, and see what you've been missing.

- **Swiss Chard Stems** - Have lots of amino acids which boost the immune system. They can be cooked in vegetable, beef or chicken stock and added to soups, broths and stews.
- **Celery Leaves** - Have more calcium and magnesium than the stalk itself. If chopped up you can add them to dips, salsa or salad.
- **Orange Peel** - Has much more fiber than the orange as well as anti-cancer and anti-inflammatory properties. It taste best when grated over foods, or dipped in (dark) chocolate. Well... everything tastes better dipped in chocolate!
- **Onion Skin** - I know this sounds crazy, but the thin skin is high in anti-oxidants. Add to your vegetable, beef or chicken stock for more flavorful soups, broths and stews.

As the saying goes "don't throw the baby out with the bath water." Enjoy your foods, but don't be so hasty to dismiss the scraps. They're good for you!

Don't Let Your Refrigerator Dictate How You Eat

Just like the strategy that grocery stores use to get you to buy certain brands of products (and yes they do this), you can change what and how much you eat by doing the same thing in the fridge. Try these tricks:

- **Nutritious food on the middle shelf** - you see it FIRST, you'll eat it first.
- **Tempting snacks are placed in opaque/dark containers** - Less likely to trigger a craving if you don't see them.
- **Do the prep for the good stuff** - Have healthy snacks ready to eat, so you can grab and go.
- **Keep the receipt on the door** - If you see what's in the fridge first and how much the good stuff cost, you may want to eat it before it goes bad.

How Do I Know When to Stop Eating?

Sometimes no matter how our food taste (good or bad), we clean our plates. Even if we're FULL. That sensation of fullness is there for a reason. The body produces certain chemicals to let you know when to put the fork down. If you choose to ignore them (like many of us do from time to time), the results are usually not pretty.

Here are a few things to pay attention to when you are eating:

- Eat slowly: The slower you eat, the less you will eat. It takes some time for the signals from the brain to come through, but you will feel full sooner and not over indulge.
- Stop eating: See how you feel. If you're honestly still hungry, go ahead and eat a little more. But if not, despite how good it looks or taste, don't do it. Push the plate

away or cover with your napkin to help you resist the temptation.

- Try to stay in range: You should always be somewhere between slightly hungry but can wait to eat, and full but not stuffed. This can be accomplished by eating small meals/snacks every 4 hours throughout the day, rather than 2 or 3 meals where you gorge yourself.

Try this method for a week or two and see how much better you feel.

Chapter Six

HOW WE EAT

In this chapter I'm describing a selection of cuisines and life-style diets that reflect ethnic, regional, cultural and ethical orientations, as well as particular beliefs about foods and their ability to support good health and heal disease.

POPULAR REGIONAL/ETHNIC CUISINES AND LIFE-STYLE DIETS

Traditional American Cuisine

Traditional American Cuisine is a mish-mash of ethnic foods imported by the many immigrants to the United States and influenced by Native American ingredients and cooking methods. That said, American food is generally characterized as some combination of meat and potatoes: hamburgers, hotdogs, ribs, steak, French fries, potato salad, mashed potatoes and potato chips, served with vegetable side-dishes such as steamed or sautéed greens, salad or corn, with apple pie or ice cream for dessert. Other dishes that are typically served in American-style restaurants include pancakes, waffles, bacon, fried eggs, bagels with cream cheese, pizza, lasagna, mac & cheese, baked beans, chili, meat loaf, fried chicken, tacos, quesadillas, sandwiches, tomato soup, clam chowder, Caesar salad, spinach salad, Cobb salad, corn bread, biscuits, fruit cobblers and pies, cakes and cookies. Fast food is also uniquely American, from McDonalds' Big Mac, to Taco Bell's Soft Taco Supreme.

Traditional American food is often thought of as "comfort" food. Comfort food is the yummy, greasy, sweet, salty, bready stuff of American childhoods. A grilled cheese sandwich with chocolate chip cookies, mac & cheese with an ice cream sundae. Delicious certainly, but healthy, not so much. Fortunately, American cuisine is ever changing and American chefs and cooks are some of the most innovative in the world. "New American Cuisine," like traditional American fare, represents a melting-pot of different cuisines from around the globe, with the difference being that New American Cuisine places an emphasis on healthy (non-GMO, pesticide free, organic), locally sourced produce, meat and fish prepared cleanly, simply and elegantly. New America Cuisine originated from what has been termed "California Cuisine," a movement started in the early 1970's at Chez Panisse restaurant in Berkeley, California by chef and restaurateur Alice Waters, who was an early advocate of sustainably grown, fresh, locally procured foods prepared with an awareness of what went into creating healthy meals. New American Cuisine has expanded to include modern, healthy interpretations of classic American fare, and reinterpretations of ethnic dishes using American ingredients.

American Regional Cuisine

California Cuisine, as discussed, got its start with Alice Waters, but was heavily influenced by Asian cuisine and chefs like Wolfgang Puck, who pioneered the "haute cuisine pizza," in his famous West Hollywood restaurant, Spago, and Jeramiah Tower, whose restaurant, Stars, in San Francisco became one of the highest grossing restaurants in the country. Why, you might ask? The food was politically correct, fresh and glamorous, but unpretentious and promoted the idea that healthy food could be more than sprouts and hummus in a pita pocket. Simply put, California Cuisine is delicious, healthy and beautifully prepared. It initiated the rise of the "celebrity chef" in American culture and is ultimately responsible for the general public's increased interest in creative food preparation and fusion cuisine.

Southwestern Cuisine is a combination of the cooking traditions of the original Spanish colonial settlers, the Native Americans indigenous to the region and later, the pioneers and cowboys who made their homes in the Southwest. That area is roughly defined as Southern California, Nevada, Arizona, New Mexico, Utah, Colorado, Oklahoma and Texas. Today, a lot of Southwestern Cuisine is similar to Mexican Cuisine and consists of dishes made from ingredients like beans, rice, corn, avocados, cheese, meat and fish, that are served with tortillas or sopaipillas, tomato salsas and sauces made from chili peppers. Each state has its own version of Southwestern or Mexican influenced cuisine, and though there are similarities, there are distinct differences from state to state. For instance, fajitas are an invention of Tex-Mex cuisine (out of Texas), and red and green chili sauce is ubiquitous in New Mexican cooking.

Southern Cuisine is derived from the culinary influences of the many different people who settled in the southern area of the United States, including Native American, African, English, Scottish, Irish, French, Spanish, Portuguese and German. Early American settlers cultivated indigenous crops such as corn, nuts, beans, squash and tomatoes and learned to barbeque from the Native Americans. They also caught fresh seafood and wild game. The Spanish introduced pigs to the area and African slaves smuggled in the seeds for okra, yams, collard greens and watermelon. Some of the dishes associated with Southern cooking include pork barbeque, fried chicken, fried catfish, shrimp gumbo, barbequed ribs, black-eyed peas, fried okra, collard greens, succotash, fried green tomatoes, corn bread, cheese grits, biscuits and gravy, fruit cobblers, pecan and sweet potato pies.

Mediterranean Cuisine

Mediterranean Cuisine represents a broad and varied conglomeration of cuisines from the countries that border the Mediterranean Sea. Although the cuisines of these different countries are often quite disparate, they have certain elements in common because of some similarities in climate and topography, as well as their proximity to the sea. The climate in the Mediterranean is generally temperate, so the entire region is blessed with an abundance of fruits and vegetables, grains, legumes and herbs, all staples of Mediterranean cuisine, no matter how differently they might be prepared from country to country.

Because of the abundance of fresh vegetables, they are often served with every meal and are generally prepared simply. Vegetables are frequently eaten in salads, or grilled, roasted, sautéed or baked, and are often prepared with olive oil, garlic and fresh herbs. Some of the most common vegetables found in the Mediterranean region are, lettuces and greens of all kinds, cucumbers, tomatoes, peas, beets, onions, leeks, carrots, squash, potatoes, peppers, artichokes, mushrooms, zucchini, eggplant, okra and broccoli.

Bread, pasta and whole grains are a mainstay in many of the region's cuisines. Whole grains and grain based foods are often cooked with meat, fish or legumes. Some of the grains used in Mediterranean cooking include wheat, rice, barley, bulgur and farro. Some of the grain based dishes you might find in a Mediterranean diet include, pastas of all kinds, grain salads, couscous, pilafs, rice dishes and risotto. A wide variety of breads from olive bread to pita bread to flat breads are an important part of most meals.

Meat is eaten sparingly, while seafood is liberally consumed. The coastal regions are too rocky for raising cattle, so smaller animals like goats, sheep, chickens and pigs are raised for meat. Cheese and yogurt is generally made from goat's milk or sheep's milk. Olives, nuts, wine grapes and fruit all thrive in the rich Mediterranean soil, so red wine in particular, olive and nut oils, whole nuts as well as fresh and dried fruits are enjoyed. Desserts are often sweetened with fresh or dried fruit, figs and honey, so the consumption of refined white sugar is kept to a minimum.

Basically, Mediterranean Cuisine is based on what's available in the region and is less processed than American food. Because the balmy climate, rich soil and sea yield a wide variety of fresh foods, the cuisine is naturally healthy. Mediterranean people traditionally spend more time luxuriating over their meals than Americans and because of this are said to have a healthier, more relaxed life-style and attitude. This may be a stereotype, but the idea that the kind of ingredients used, along with specific methods of food preparation and the way meals are savored and enjoyed, could promote greater health and longevity, captured the imagination of the American people over fifty years ago.

The "Mediterranean Diet" refers to a modern adaptation of the traditional cuisines of the Mediterranean for the purposes of creating and maintaining good health. The diet has been of particular interest to those concerned with cardiovascular health and longevity. There have been studies that correlate general good health, heart health and longer life spans with the Mediterranean diet. In the West, it is thought that the main components of the diet that confer good health are the consumption of large quantities of fresh vegetables and fruits, the liberal use of olive oil in salads and in cooking, the moderate to low consumption of red meat and dairy, and the enthusiastic enjoyment of red wine.

Vegetarian / Vegan Cuisine

Vegetarians do not eat meat and some abstain from eating eggs, dairy, seafood and animal by-products (which are often found in packaged and pre-prepared foods). This diet is often a life-style choice having as much do with health considerations as with moral, ethical or religious considerations. Many vegetarians believe that a meatless diet is healthier, and there is evidence supporting the fact that less or no meat – provided the diet includes a viable source of protein – can decrease the incidence of certain diseases, like cardiovascular disease, cancer and diabetes.

Some vegetarians are morally opposed to killing sentient beings, others abstain due to religious beliefs and still others are opposed to the cruel treatment of animals bred for slaughter, as well as the damage that the meat industry allegedly does to the environment. Of course there are some people who just simply don't like the taste of meat. This is a diet that can be challenging to sustain, unless you have some awareness of nutrition. It's important to make sure you get enough protein in your diet if you are not eating meat. Some complete proteins that are good substitutes for meat are, rice and beans, quinoa, and soy.

Vegans are very strict vegetarians with a moral basis for their diet and life-style. They don't eat meat, eggs, dairy, seafood or anything processed using animal products like white sugar or anything produced by animals like honey. Donald Watson coined the term vegan in 1944, and defined it as follows: "Veganism is a way of living which excludes all forms of exploitation of, and cruelty to, the animal kingdom, and includes a reverence for life. It applies to the practice of living on the products of the plant kingdom to the exclusion of flesh, fish, fowl, eggs, honey, animal milk and its derivatives, and encourages the use of alternatives for all commodities derived wholly or in part from animals."

A few of my clients who have decided on the vegan lifestyle ask about calcium. How will I get enough? Am I more prone to break a bone without calcium in my diet? Fortunately for them, nature has taken care of this problem. There are multiple (non-dairy) sources from which to choose. For example, soy milk! Yes it's not much, but there is calcium in it. Nuts and seeds like flax and sesame and multiple veggies, especially the DARK greens, like spinach, kale, collards, and broccoli are always a good source.

China Study

The China Study diet is based on a book published in 2005 called *The China Study: Startling Implications for Diet, Weight Loss and Long-term Health*, by biochemist, T. Colin Campbell, PhD, and his son, Thomas M. Campbell II, MD. T. Colin Campbell is featured in the 2011 American documentary film, *Forks over Knives*, which provides an overview of the research study (China-Oxford-Cornell Project) that led to his book. Very simply put, the diet the Campbells advocate, based on many years of research, is a whole foods, plant-based diet.

T. Colin Campbell was one of the directors of the 20-year study called The China-Oxford-Cornell Project. The results of the study showed that people who eat primarily a whole-foods, plant-based diet live longer, healthier lives than those who eat a diet high in animal proteins. People who eat meat and processed foods were shown to suffer from a greater incidence of certain cancers, coronary disease, obesity, diabetes and other chronic diseases. Sanjay Gupta, Chief Medical Correspondent for CNN, stated that the diet changed the way he eats, and former President Bill Clinton credits the diet for his significant weight loss in 2010.

Chapter Eleven (p. 225-240) in *The China Study* outlines its eight principles of food and health. Principle #1: "Nutrition represents the combined activities of countless food substances. The whole is greater than the sum of its parts." In other words, variety is one of the keys to good nutrition. Nutrients in your food work together and it's a mistake to think one specific nutrient is going to make you healthy or solve your health problems. Principle #2: "Vitamin supplements are not a panacea for good health." Consuming isolated nutrients in the form of supplements cannot take the place of consuming a rich variety of whole foods. Only the nutrients found in whole foods are truly beneficial to the body. Principle #3: "There are virtually no nutrients in animal-based foods that are not better provided by plants." Principle #4: "Genes do not determine disease on their own. Genes function only by being activated, or expressed, and nutrition plays a critical role in determining which genes, good and bad, are expressed." Principle #5: "Nutrition can substantially control the adverse effects of noxious chemicals." The nutrient imbalances that animal-based and processed foods create within the body are more responsible for disease than the toxic chemicals we are exposed to in our environment or food. Principle #6: "The same nutrition that prevents disease in its early stages (before diagnosis) can also halt or reverse disease in its later stages (after diagnosis)." The nutrition being touted by the Study derives from plant-based, whole foods. Principle #7: "Nutrition that is truly beneficial for one chronic disease will support health across the board." And finally,

Principle #8: "Good nutrition creates health in all areas of our existence. All parts are interconnected."

So what exactly does this diet consist of? As much as you want of a good variety of any whole, unrefined plant-based food - fruits; vegetables, including roots, legumes, and mushrooms; nuts; whole grains, including rice, quinoa, wheat, millet, oats, buckwheat, spelt, corn, rye, kamut, sorghum, barley, teff and amaranth. Eat only a minimal amount of refined carbohydrates (white flour and sugar), vegetable oils (corn, olive and peanut), and fish. Avoid completely, meat, poultry, dairy and eggs. In spite of the admonition that supplements can't take the place of a well-rounded, whole-food, plant-based meal, the Campbells recommend supplementing with vitamin B12 (naturally found in meat, fish, eggs and dairy) and vitamin D (naturally found in fatty fish and egg yolks). Vitamin D is produced in the body when the sun's rays hit bare skin, so you don't have to supplement with vitamin D if you get enough sun exposure.

Raw Food Diet and Juicing

The Raw Food Diet advocates eating all food raw and unprocessed, including meat, fish and dairy. The exception to this rule is that it's okay to heat food as long as it is not heated over 118 degrees Fahrenheit. The theory behind this diet is that excessive heat destroys valuable enzymes and nutrients in food. Although there are adherents of this diet who eat raw meat, dairy and fish, the mainstay of the diet is fruits, vegetables, nuts and seeds. The diet is said to cure a host of diseases, and proponents of the diet say that they feel better, have more energy, are able to lose weight, look younger and are happier on the diet.

Although the diet may seem limited and boring at first, those who have adopted it with enthusiasm employ their creativity in creating meals that are more than just salads or smoothies. There are recipes available online and a large selection of raw food "cook" books available for those who want to explore the myriad options for creating interesting meals with raw food.

Juicing has become wildly popular of late. By putting fresh vegetables and fruits through an electric juicer, a concentrated, highly nutritious liquid is extracted. Juicing leaves most of the fiber behind, which makes the juice easier for the body to digest and the nutrients easier for it to absorb. The quality of the juice will have a lot to do with the kind of juicer used. The highest quality juicers can produce juice that will hold its nutritional value for up to three days if stored in the refrigerator in a tightly sealed container. Juicers that cause more oxidation by grinding up or heating the vegetables and fruits produce juice that must be consumed immediately to receive the full benefit of the vitamins, minerals, antioxidants and enzymes in the vegetables and fruits. The types of vegetables and fruits juiced have a huge impact on the benefits you'll receive. Most people who drink fresh juice, advocate juicing mainly vegetables rather than fruit, in order to avoid consuming too much sugar.

Proponents of juicing feel that the concentration of natural nutrients in fresh juices are easier for the body to absorb and utilize than the nutrients in vitamin or mineral pills. They claim that adding fresh juice to the diet can help regulate weight, strengthen immunity, improve energy levels and detox the body. There are those who believe that drinking fresh juice on a regular basis and/or doing periodic or long-term cleanses can reduce the incidence of cancer and heart disease and even cure certain diseases.

Doing cleanses with fresh juices in which nothing but juice is consumed for several days or longer can cause some people, particularly those who aren't used to periodic cleansing, to feel sick. During cleanses, the body can detox too quickly and cause flu-like symptoms and fatigue. There has also been some concern that avid juicers are drinking too much kale and spinach, which can cause a surplus of oxalic acid in the body, which in turn can lead to thyroid and hormonal issues. It's best to mix it up by juicing a wide variety of vegetables with only a small amount of fruits in order to get a balanced and complete supply of nutrients.

Paleo Diet

Though the modern Paleo diet has been kicking around since the 1970's, its most prominent, recent advocate is university professor, Loren Cordain, who has written a series of books on the Paleo diet. The Paleo or Paleolithic Diet (also known as the Caveman Diet) is based on the idea that from a genetic point of view, we humans haven't evolved significantly beyond our Stone Age ancestors and therefore are more adapted to eat what they presumably ate, than the highly processed, carb heavy food we eat now. Proponents of the Paleo diet claim that it can reduce the incidence of diseases associated with the consumption of highly processed foods, particularly heart disease, obesity and diabetes.

The agricultural revolution was only 10,000 years ago and marked the end of the Paleolithic era. Since that time, humans have incorporated grain into what was formerly a hunter-gatherer diet, consisting of fish, meat, eggs, fruits, vegetables, leafy greens, nuts, seeds, roots, mushrooms, herbs and spices. The modern adaptation of the Paleolithic diet, includes all the "hunter-gather" foods as well as healthy oils (olive, coconut, avocado), and eliminates all processed foods, grains, dairy, legumes, refined sugar, salt, refined vegetable oils and alcohol. If you can't eat wild game on a regular basis, the diet advocates the consumption of organic, grass-fed, free-range meat, and instead of fruits and vegetables from Mexico or South America or even from across the country, only locally sourced, seasonal fruits and veggies.

Ayurvedic Cuisine

Ayurveda is an ancient, traditional Hindu healing system that focuses on the mind-body connection. Diet is just one of the many healing approaches used in Ayurveda. In addition to specific dietary recommendations, Ayurvedic treatment might include detoxification through fasting and body treatments, herbal medicine, massage, yoga and meditation. The diet is based in part on the theory of body types and their relationship to the five elements – fire, water, earth, air and space. In Ayurveda, there are three distinct body-types or "doshas," and most people are a combination of two, but there is generally one that will define a person's dominant characteristics and ultimately determine the kind of diet and course of treatment to be prescribed.

The three doshas are Vata, Pitta and Kapha. An Ayurvedic practitioner can identify your dosha, or you can answer a series of questions (found online) that will help you determine your predominant type. Vata dosha consists of air and space elements. Vata people are energetic, enthusiastic, quick learners, creative and naturally slender. They have a tendency to be cold and often have dry hair and skin. If the Vata individual is out of balance, he or she may experience anxiety and insomnia. Pitta dosha consists of fire and water elements. The Pitta person tends to be intense, passionate, smart and enterprising with a medium build and good muscle tone. Out of balance, the Pitta person will express anger or irritation, have digestive problems and be prone to overwork. Kapha dosha consists of earth and water elements. The Kapha person tends to be physically larger and strong with thick, wavy hair. He or she also tends to be loyal and sensual. When out of balance, the Kapha person can become resistant to change and might manifest allergies and suffer from sluggish digestion which can lead to weight gain and even obesity.

The Ayurvedic diet consists of six tastes: sweet, sour, salty, bitter, pungent and astringent. If all six tastes are included in every meal, you can be sure you are getting all the nutrients you need and that you will feel satiated. Each taste represents a group of specific foods. Once you or your practitioner has determined your dosha, you can begin modifying your diet to accommodate your type, which will help you stay in balance, give you energy, curb cravings, stabilize your weight and regulate your moods.

One dietary recommendation to keep the Vata dosha in balance is to eat warm, cooked foods and vegetables especially ones that are salty, sweet or sour. In the Ayurvedic system, salty foods include fish and seaweed, sweet foods include meat, whole grains and dairy, and sour foods include tomatoes, cheese and berries among many other foods. The Vata dosha is encouraged to minimize his or her intake of foods that are bitter, astringent or pungent. Bitter foods include, spinach, kale, leafy greens and broccoli, astringent foods include lentils, cauliflower and figs, and pungent foods include salsa, ginger and onions. (The entire list of foods associated with the tastes is available online or in any number of good books on Ayurveda.) The Pitta person is encouraged to eat cool foods and liquids, favor the sweet, bitter and astringent tastes and minimize foods that are salty, pungent or sour. The Kapha dosha is advised to eat a lot of vegetables and spices, to favor bitter, pungent or astringent tastes and minimize foods that are salty, sour or sweet.

You can see that this is not a simple diet, and to be truly effective is best prescribed by a trained Ayurvedic practitioner. Although you can prepare the recommended foods as you wish, the traditional recipes for Ayurvedic food employ the cooking practices, food combinations and spices of the broader Indian cuisine.

Gluten-Free Diet

A gluten-free diet is mandatory for people with celiac disease and good for people with a sensitivity to gluten. Celiac disease is an autoimmune disease that affects the digestive system. When a person with celiac disease eats gluten (a protein found in wheat, rye and barley), the immune system attacks the villi in the small intestine, which prevents the absorption of nutrients into the body. Many people who do not have celiac disease have a sensitivity to gluten and experience uncomfortable symptoms when they eat products continuing gluten. Some of the more common symptoms of gluten sensitivity are rashes, digestive problems, joint pain and fatigue.

The gluten-free diet is quite straight-forward and requires only that you recognize the foods you must avoid. Obviously wheat, barley and rye are no-no's. Many packaged and pre-prepared foods have gluten added, so it's important to check labels and ingredient lists and only buy packaged foods that are labeled "gluten-free." It is also important to be alert to the possibility of cross-contamination. Some products that are gluten-free are manufactured in plants that also manufacture products containing gluten. Manufacturers are not obligated to state this on packaging.

Chapter Seven

WHAT HAVE YOU TRIED IN THE PAST?

In order to give you a clear, concise and comprehensive idea of what's available to you in the land of diet plans, I am providing you with descriptions of the most popular diets from the past fifty years. I'm sure you have tried one or two or all of them in the past with limited or no success. In my opinion pre-packaged, highly processed foods are not the best option for optimal health. Most of them contain excess amounts of sugar, salt and fat, and none of those things support your quest for getting healthy and feeing better. Eating is something we all must do to survive, but should it be this hard? Should it require counting points, measuring or having limited choices as to what you can eat?

MEAL REPLACEMENT DIET PLANS:

Medifast Diet Plan

The Medifast Diet Plan is a meal replacement plan that was introduced to the public in 1980. The diet was developed by a doctor and the products were originally only available through a doctor's office and required a prescription. The products are now available through the company's website. The most widely used Medifast diet plan, called the Medifast 5 & 1 Plan, can be self-monitored or overseen by a professional at a Medifast Weight Control Center, by a Medifast sanctioned Health Coach or by any doctor who distributes the products.

The Medifast 5 & 1 Plan consists of five meal replacement products, plus one "Lean & Green Meal" per day, prepared according to Medifast instructions. The five Medifast meals can be any one of their more than 70 meal replacement products. There are three "Phases" to the Meal Plan. Phase One is the basic diet as described so far, and is meant to last for as long as it takes you to reach your weight-loss goal. Phase Two is the transition plan, which allows you to gradually increase the amount of calories you're eating by adding back in different foods each week for six weeks. Phase Three is the maintenance plan, which is individually formulated for each person.

Slimfast

Slimfast, like Medifast, is a meal replacement plan. The first Slimfast meal replacement shakes were made available to the public in 1977. Between then and now, the company has developed a variety of different meal replacement products, but they are currently only selling their 3-2-1 line of products. The Slimfast 3-2-1 Plan is an easy and flexible daily diet plan described in detail on the Slimfast website. The daily meal consists of three Slimfast snack bars, snack bites or fruits and vegetables of your choice, two Slimfast Protein Shakes or Meal Bars and one "sensible" 500 calorie meal of your choice. The website suggests that a sensible, balanced meal consists of half a plate of vegetables, a quarter of a plate of lean protein and a quarter of a plate of starch.

Slimfast claims that if you follow their diet plan you can lose up to 1-2 pounds per week. The Slimfast 3-2-1 Plan, like the Medifast Diet Plan, relies on calorie restriction to help you lose weight.

PRE-PACKAGED DIET PLANS:

Nutrisystem

Nutrisystem was founded in 1972 and has gone through a number of different incarnations since then. Today Nutrisystem offers a variety of weight loss programs tailored to women, men, people with pre-diabetes or diabetes, vegetarians, teens and people concerned with heart health. The Nutrisystem programs offer a wide selection of complete prepackaged meals - breakfasts, lunches and dinners - as well as snacks and desserts specifically organized to meet the nutritional and weight loss requirements of their target group. The meal choices are extensive (over 150 entrees) and you have the option to choose your entrees, which consist of dishes such as Apple

Cinnamon Oatmeal or Pancakes for breakfast, and Cajun-style Chicken and Sausage or Hearty Beef Stew for dinner.

The prepackaged meals eaten with the recommended additional fruits, vegetables, protein and dairy, amount to approximately 1200 calories a day for women and 1500 calories a day for men. The company claims that it is possible to lose 1-2 pounds a week on their diet and offers, in addition to the pre-prepared meals, a grocery guide; a 13-week, and self-guided, behavioral modification

Jenny Craig

Jenny Craig was founded in Australia in 1983 and moved its operations to the United States in 1985. The Jenny Craig program is somewhat similar to the Nutrisystem plan with the exception that along with the pre-packaged meals, Jenny Craig offers one-on-one, weekly nutritional and motivational counseling, and tailors its diet plan to meet the individual needs of its clients. The counseling can take place "At Home" or "In Center." If you choose the "At Home" option, you will have the opportunity to speak to your counselor once a week on the phone and have your meals delivered to your door. If you choose the "In Center" option, you will see your counselor in person once a week and pick up your meals at that time.

Although the mainstay of the Jenny Craig diet plan are the pre-packaged meals, like Nutrisystem, the program requires that the meals be supplemented with fresh fruits, vegetables and non-fat dairy products. Program participants can stay on the Jenny Craig diet for as long as they need to in order to reach their weight-loss goals. The daily diet consists of three pre-packaged meals and one snack in addition to two or three servings of non-fat dairy, fresh vegetables or fruit. Also like Nutrisystem, Jenny Craig offers a wide variety of meals, including a Cheddar Cheese Omelet or Florentine Breakfast Pizzas for breakfast, a Meatball Stuffed Sandwich for lunch, Roasted Turkey Medallions for dinner and Chocolate Walnut Brownies for dessert.

After you have gotten half way to your weight loss goal, Jenny Craig begins to wean you off the pre-packaged meals by having you prepare meals for yourself (using their recipes) two days a week. After you reach your weight loss goal, the program gives you four weeks to transition from the pre-packaged meals to dishes you prepare for yourself.

Weight Watchers

Founded in 1963, Weight Watchers is undoubtedly one of the most well-known weight loss programs in the world. It is unique in that it is the only diet plan listed here that does not offer pre-packaged/replacement meals or promote a specific type of diet. Instead it uses a point system (PointsPlus plan) that denotes the calorie content and nutritional value of food. Dieters are evaluated according to weight, height, age and gender and are then assigned a certain number of points per day and some extra per week (equal to at least 1200 calories a day) that they can "spend" on any food they want to eat.

Though it's true that participants may eat anything they want, the points system is designed to encourage healthy choices. You spend less points on food that is low in calories, fat and sugar, but rich in nutritional value. Fresh fruits and vegetables points are free, specifically to encourage dieters to eat more of these filling, nutritionally beneficial foods. Exercise is encouraged and extra points can be earned engaging in more traditional exercise such as bike riding, hiking and swimming as well as in physical activities that aren't considered "exercise," but that expend energy, such as cleaning the house and dancing the night away at a club.

One of the hallmarks of the Weight Watchers program is the community support system (in person meetings and online support forums) available to all participants. Weight Watchers claims that dieters who attend meetings regularly, lose more weight than those who go it alone. The meetings provide a place for participants to share their stories, support and encourage each other, receive guidance and motivation, and check their weight in a private ritual called the "weigh-in." Whether you choose to participate in the program by attending meetings, or taking advantage of the online support system, once you have paid the fees, you will receive support materials and tools.

HIGH PROTEIN DIETS:

The Atkins Diet

The Atkins Nutritional Approach (as it is officially called) was developed by the American cardiologist, Dr. Robert Atkins, and was introduced to the general public through his first book *Dr. Atkins' Diet Revolution*, originally published in 1972. He updated his diet (but did not change any of his core concepts) in the book *Dr. Atkins' New Diet Revolution*, published in 2002. The latest iteration of the Atkins' diet is available in a book published in 2010, entitled *The New Atkins for a New You,* by Dr. Eric C. Westman, M.D.; Dr. Stephen D. Phinney, M.D. and Dr. Jeff S. Volek, PhD. The latest version of the diet remains essentially the same as the original, except that it incorporates the latest scientific findings about nutrition made in the last ten years.

The Atkins' Diet severely restricts the consumption of carbohydrates and promotes the consumption of proteins and healthy fats. The concept is based on the fact that the body will burn stored body fat when it is starved of carbohydrates and sugars, thus hastening weight-loss. The Atkins' Diet has four phases. Phase One is referred to the Induction Phase, during which Atkins claims that you can lose up to 15 pounds in the first two weeks. You are instructed to eat 3 regular-size meals or 4-5 smaller meals without going for more than 6 waking hours without eating. Each meal should consist only of foods from the "Acceptable Foods List for Phase 1" (found on the website). Phase Two is the Ongoing Weight Loss Phase, during which you are allowed to start adding more carbs and other Atkins sanctioned foods back into your diet. If you are continuing to lose weight in this phase, you may feel you're ready to move to the next phase when you are approximately 10 pounds away from your desired weight. During Phase Three or the Pre-Maintenance Phase, you are allowed to continue adding carbs and other foods from the Atkins list. You will want to stay in this phase until you reach your weight loss goal, at which point you can transition to Phase Four - the final phase - where you establish your permanent "Lifetime Maintenance" diet plan.

Your "Lifetime Maintenance" diet will still be restricted, but much expanded from the initial phases of the diet. A brief discussion of the importance of exercise is brought up in this phase, but there is no specific exercise plan in place. The website provides recipes, an explanation of the science behind the diet, tools such as the Carb Counter and a mobile app, blogs and community forums for support and information.

The South Beach Diet

The South Beach Diet has a lot in common with the Atkins Diet including the fact that it was pioneered by a cardiologist. In an effort to help his cardiac patients prevent heart attacks and strokes, Dr. Arthur Agatston, M.D., developed the South Beach Diet and subsequently wrote a number of books about his diet plan and approach to wellness. *The South Beach Diet: The Delicious, Doctor-Designed, Foolproof Plan for Fast and Healthy Weight Loss* (published in 2003) and *The South Beach Diet Supercharged* (published in 2009) have become best sellers and mainstays in the pantheon of modern approaches to weight loss and healthy living. In addition to these books, he has written quite a few other books including cookbooks and a dining guide. He produced a workout DVD in 2008.

The South Beach Diet is essentially a low carb, high protein diet. It differs from the Atkins Diet in that it allows a greater selection of carbs from the very beginning and recommends a more limited selection of dietary fats. Unlike the Atkins Diet, The South Beach Diet ultimately weans its followers off the diet completely. The diet plan has three phases – Phase One is intended to "jump start" your weight loss, Phase Two is intended to help you reach your weight loss goal and learn healthy eating strategies in the process, and Phase Three is intended to be the maintenance phase, in which you become fully responsible for monitoring your food intake without the benefit of a strict diet plan.

During Phase One the daily diet consists of three meals featuring lean proteins, two snacks and one protein-rich dessert (something with cream and/or nuts). This diet strategy is designed to stabilize blood sugar, eliminate cravings and produce rapid weight loss in only two weeks. *The South Beach Diet Supercharged* offers a complete list of all the foods that are allowed during the three different phases. Phase Two allows you to add in "good" carbohydrates, such as fruits, whole grains and additional vegetables. You will stay in Phase Two for as long as it takes you to reach your weight loss goal. After you have reached your goal, you move to Phase Three, where you will learn to maintain your weight. During this phase, you will be able to eat any food you want because in theory you have learned through the course of the diet how to make healthy food choices and how to eat in moderation.

NEW KIDS ON THE BLOCK:

<u>The Shred Diet</u>

The Shred Diet was developed by Dr. Ian Smith, M.D., who has made appearances on a number of TV shows including *VH1's Celebrity Fit Club*, and *The Dr. Oz Show*. In 2007, he initiated a national campaign called the "50 Million Pound Challenge" to inspire people to get healthy by losing weight and getting in shape. His book, *Shred: The Revolutionary Diet* was published in December 2012. He developed the diet specifically to help people who felt they had reached a plateau in their weight loss programs or felt they couldn't find a diet plan that truly worked for them. The Shred Diet is predicated on a theory originated by Dr. Ian, which he calls "Diet Confusion." Diet Confusion was inspired by the idea of muscle confusion. By constantly varying your diet you trick your body out of its stable metabolic rhythm and cause the metabolism to speed up in the same way that muscle confusion tricks complacent muscles into developing. When the metabolism speeds up, the body burns fat and releases weight more quickly and efficiently.

The diet is very specific and takes you through a strict six week protocol. The book claims that "Shredders" lose on the average 20 pounds, 2 sizes or 4 inches by the end of the six week program. The food on the diet plan is low on the glycemic index, so it keeps blood sugar levels stable, which will help you feel more satiated and boost your energy level. The plan also employs meal spacing and uses meal replacements both of which curb hunger cravings and speed weight loss. The Shred weight loss plan includes a workout schedule with a variety of exercise options.

The diet program takes you week by week through different phases and includes a comprehensive list of the foods you can eat and a time table for eating them. The phases, which each last one week, are: Prime, Challenge, Transformation, Ascend, Cleanse, and Explode. Each phase has different rules and different combinations of meals and meal replacements. The phases are structured to build on each other and the program is designed to ease you into the diet. The meals are laid out in detail, so you don't have to think too much about what to eat, but all the meals are comprised of "normal," affordable foods.

The 100 Diet

In May of 2013, diet and weight loss expert Jorge Cruise published his latest diet book: *The 100: Count Only Sugar Calories and Lose Up to 18 Lbs. in Two Weeks.* He developed The 100 Diet based on his understanding of the most cutting edge science behind weight loss. He claims that sugar calories are the only calories that count, and that the conventional wisdom that claims weight loss is determined by the number of calories in versus the number of calories out is inaccurate. His diet, in essence, is exceedingly simple. Restrict consumption of sugar calories to less than 100 a day, and you will lose weight – guaranteed. The book claims (in its title, no less) that if you stick to his 4-week program you can lose as much as 18 pounds within the first 2 weeks and 2 pounds a week thereafter.

The science behind his sugar-calories-are-the-only-calories-that-count concept is that insulin regulates fat storage in the body and carbohydrate consumption causes insulin secretion. The more carbohydrates we consume, the more insulin we secrete, the more fat we store. Cruise gives a simple formula for calculating the number of sugar calories for all carbohydrates and his book lists many carbohydrates with their corresponding sugar calories. If you want to eat something that's not listed in his book, you will have to consult the internet for carbohydrate information, or if you are eating a packaged food item, you can consult the nutritional information on the package.

EPILOGUE

Now it's time for you to make a few decisions. How do you want to live? What do you want to do and how do you want to feel with the time you have left?

This book is the blue print for your new life plan:

- The WHO - You.
- The WHAT - Change what you feed your mind and body.
- The WHEN - Right now.
- The WHERE - Start at home and take changes to the office.
- The HOW - Replace one food at a time.
- The WHY - Because your life depends on it.

I'm here to support you so... let's go!!

APPENDIX A

DEFINITIONS

Antioxidant - Substances that inhibit oxidation (deterioration due to exposure to oxygen).

Artificial Sweeteners - Synthetic sugar substitutes that mimic the taste of sugar such as aspartame (NutraSweet, Equal), saccharine (Sweet 'N Low) and sucralose (Splenda).

Body Mass Index (BMI) – This measure is used as a way to assess how much a person's weight conforms to what is considered to be normal for their height. It is often used to determine whether someone is under or overweight or obese. It is the measure of weight in kilograms divided by height in meters squared.

Cage Free/Free Range - Poultry raised in an outdoor setting, roaming uncaged.

Carbohydrate – A nutrient that comes in the form of sugars (found in honey, fruits, vegetables and dairy products) and starches (found in potatoes, corn and wheat).

Dietary Fat – A nutrient that is generally insoluble in water, mainly characterized as saturated or unsaturated (found in meats, dairy, eggs, nuts and seeds).

Fat Free – On food labels: less than 0.5 grams of fat per serving.

GMO - Genetically Modified Organisms.

Gluten - A protein with an elastic texture found in wheat, barley and rye.

Glycemic Index - Ranks carbohydrates on a scale from 0 to 100, according to their effect on blood sugar levels in the body.

Glycemic Load - Accounts for how much each gram of carbohydrate in food raises blood sugar levels. Based on the glycemic index.

Grass Fed - Refers to beef, goats and sheep that have been raised on only grass and mothers milk.

Natural – According to the USDA: "A product containing no artificial ingredient or added color and is only minimally processed. Minimal processing means that the product was processed in a manner that does not fundamentally alter the product. The label must include a statement explaining the meaning of the term natural (such as 'no artificial ingredients; minimally processed')."

Nutrient Dense – According to the Dietary Guidelines for Americans 2005: foods that provide substantial amounts of vitamins and minerals and relatively few calories.

Obese - An excess of adipose tissues (body fat) and a BMI of 30-39.9 kilograms/meters squared.

Organic – Animals (cattle, dairy cows, poultry, pigs and sheep) that are not given antibiotics or hormones, or fed non-organic feed. Non-GMO vegetables and fruits that are not sprayed with chemical herbicides or pesticides.

Overweight - A BMI of 25-29 kilograms/meter squared.

Protein - An essential nutrient made up of amino acids. Foods that contain all nine essential amino acids are called complete proteins (beef, chicken, fish, eggs, milk and soybeans).

Sugar (different names) - barley malt, cane-juice crystals, caramel, carob syrup, corn sweetener, corn syrup, corn syrup solids, dextran, dextrose, fructose, fruit juice, glucose, high-fructose corn syrup or HFCS, honey, juice, lactose, malt syrup, maltodextrin, maltose, mannitol, maple syrup, molasses, sorbitol, sorghum syrup, sucrose, syrup.

Whole Foods – Foods that have not been processed and have had no artificial substances added to them.

Whole Grains – Grains that have not been broken down or processed so they retain all their nutrients and fiber.

APPENDIX B

NUTRITIONAL CONTENT OF
POPULAR FAST FOOD MEALS

FAST FOOD CHAIN	FOOD	CALORIES	FAT GRAMS
BURGER KING	Whopper	670	39
	Whopper w/cheese	760	47
	French Fries (medium)	360	20
	Onion Rings (medium)	310	15
KFC	Chicken Breast,	380	19
	Original	460	28
	Chicken Breast, Extra	140	8
	Crunchy	120	4
	Drumstick, Original	180	11
	Mashed Potatoes w/		
	gravy		
	Coleslaw		
MCDONALD'S	Big Mac	560	30
	Quarter Pounder	420	18
	Double Quarter	980	62
	Pounder w/cheese	420	9
	Chicken McNuggets (6)	380	20
	Premium Grilled	270	12
	Chicken Classic	330	8
	French Fries (medium)	340	10
	Apple Pie		
	Hot Fudge Sundae		

PIZZA HUT	Cheese Pizza Pan Pizza (2 slices) Cheese Pizza Thin 'N Crispy (2 slices) Pepperoni Pizza Pan Pizza Pepperoni Pizza Thin 'N Crispy	560 400 580 420	26 16 30 20
SUBWAY	6 inch Turkey Breast Sub 6 inch Club w/turkey, ham, roast beef 6 inch Meatball Marinara Chocolate Chip Cookie Peanut Butter Cookie	280 320 560 210 220	4.5 6 24 10 12
TACO BELL	Bean Burrito Burrito Supreme w/ steak Burrito Supreme Fresco Style Taco, Crunchy Taco, Soft Cinnamon Twists Nachos	370 420 350 170 200 170 330	10 16 9 10 9 7 21
WENDY'S	Big Bacon Classic Ultimate Chicken Grill Sandwich Chicken Nuggets (5) French Fries (medium) Large Chili	580 360 230 430 330	29 7 15 20 9
CHIPOTLE	Chicken Burrito Steak Burrito 3 Chicken Tacos, Soft 3 Chicken Tacos, Hard 3 Steak Tacos, Soft 3 Steak Tacos, Hard	1043 1033 710 635 700 625	40 40 34 33 34 33

REFERENCES

Chapter One - *The Mysterious Ways of the Food Industry*

Campbell, T. Colin, and Thomas M. Campbell II. *The China Study: Startling Implications for Diet, Weight Loss and Long-term Health*. Dallas: BenBella Books, 2006. Print.

Cummins, Ronnie. "How Factory Farming Contributes to Global Warming." *ecowatch.com*, Eco Watch. January 21, 2013. Web.

"Food Guide Pyramid." *wikipedia.org*. Web.

Hartwig, Dallas, and Melissa Hartwig. *It Starts with Food: Discover the Whole30 and Change Your Life in Unexpected Ways*. Las Vegas: Victory Belt Publishing, 2012. Print.

"Monsanto: A Corporate Profile." *foodandwaterwatch.org*, Food and Water Watch. August 8, 2013. Web.

Moss, Michael. *Salt Sugar Fat: How the Food Giants Hooked Us*. New York: Random House, 2013. Print.

"Obesity and Overweight (Data are for the U.S.)." *cdc.gov*, Centers for Disease Control and Prevention. November 21, 2013. Web.

Smith, Jeffrey M. "Doctors Warn: Avoid Genetically Modified Food." *responsibletechnology.com*, Institute for Responsible Technology. May 2009. Web.

"U.S. and Monsanto Dominate Global Market for GM Seeds." *organicconsumers.org*, Organic Consumers Association. August 7, 2013. Web.

Whitman, Deborah B. "Genetically Modified Foods: Harmful or Helpful?" *csa.com*. April 2000. Web.

Chapter Two - *Why It Matters What You Eat*

Babal, Ken. "The Best Colon-Cleansing Diet." *alive.com*, Alive. August 2002. Web.

"Brain." *wikipedia.org*. Web.

Brain, Marshall. "How Sunburns and Sun Tans Work." *howstuffworks.com*, How Stuff Works. Web.

Callahan, Maureen. "Fiftysomething Diet: Eating Habits That Hurt Your Liver." *nextavenue.org*, Next Avenue. February 15, 2013. Web.

"Colon." *wikipedia.org*. Web.

Dachis, Adam. "What Sugar Actually Does to Your Brain and Body." *lifehacker.com*, Life Hacker. June 7, 2011. Web.

Editorial Team. "Why Is Alcohol Bad for Your Liver?" *thehealthsite.com*, The Health Site. Web.

"Heart." *wikipedia.org*. Web.

Henderson, Roger. "How the Heart Works." *netdoctor.co.uk*, Net Doctor. Web.

"Kidney." *wikipedia.org*. Web.

"The Kidneys and How They Work." *kidney.niddk.nih.gov*, US Department of Health and Human Services. February 2014. Web.

Kinser, Patricia Anne. "Comparative Neuroanatomy and Intelligence." *serendip.brynmawr.edu*, Serendip Studio. December 2000. Web.

Lewis, Tanya. "Human Heart: Anatomy, Function & Facts." *livescience.com*, Live Science. May 23, 2013. Web.

Mehdi. "20 Super Foods You Need to Build Muscle & Lose Fat." *stronglifts.com*, Stronglifts. June 18, 2008. Web.

"Muscle." *wikipedia.org*. Web.

Nordqvist, Christian. "What Is Heart Disease." *medicalnewstoday.com*, Medical News Today. November 5, 2011. Web.

Oz, Mehmet. "What Does the Liver Do?" *oprah.com*, Oprah. August 19, 2008. Web.

"The Pancreas." *pathology.jhu.edu*, Johns Hopkins Medicine. Web.

Patel, Arti. "Foods for Liver: 10 Foods for a Health and Clean Liver." *huffingtonpost.ca*, Huffpost Living Canada. September 13, 2012. Web.

Sorgen, Carol. "Eat Smart for a Healthier Brain." *webmd.com*, Web MD. Web.

Taylor, Tim. "Liver." *innerbody.com*, Inner Body. Web.

"Top 10 Ways to Protect Your Liver." *cncahealth.com*, CNCA Health. Web.

"Type 2 Diabetes Overview." *webmd.com*, Web MD. 2012. Web.

"Understanding Kidney Disease – Symptoms." *webmd.com*, Web MD. Web.

Wheldon, Julie. "Too Much Junk Food Does Clog the Brain." dailymail.co.uk, Mail Online. April 16, 2005. Web.

Chapter Three - *How Primary Foods Affect What You Eat*

Rosenthal, Joshua. *Integrative Nutrition: Feed Your Hunger for Health and Happiness.* Integrative Nutrition Publishing, February 18, 2014 (Third Edition). Print.

Chapter Four - *Yes, There Is Another Way and It's Not a Diet!*

Colbin, Annemarie. *Food and Healing.* Ballantine Books, July 12, 1986 (Paperback reissue). Print.

Hartwig, Dallas, and Melissa Hartwig. *It Starts with Food: Discover the Whole30 and Change Your Life in Unexpected Ways.* Las Vegas: Victory Belt Publishing, 2012. Print.

Nestle, Marion. *What to Eat.* North Point Press, May 2, 2006. Print

Rosenthal, Joshua. *Integrative Nutrition: Feed Your Hunger for Health and Happiness.* Integrative Nutrition Publishing, February 18, 2014 (Third Edition). Print.

Chapter Five - *Staying on Track*

Colbin, Annemarie. *Food and Healing*. Ballantine Books, July 12, 1986 (Paperback reissue). Print.

Hartwig, Dallas, and Melissa Hartwig. *It Starts with Food: Discover the Whole30 and Change Your Life in Unexpected Ways*. Las Vegas: Victory Belt Publishing, 2012. Print.

Nestle, Marion. *What to Eat*. North Point Press, May 2, 2006. Print

Rosenthal, Joshua. *Integrative Nutrition: Feed Your Hunger for Health and Happiness*. Integrative Nutrition Publishing, February 18, 2014 (Third Edition). Print.

Chapter Six - *How We Eat*

"American Cuisine: New American." *mygourmetconnection. com*, My Gourmet Connection. Web.

"The Beginner's Guide to the Paleo Diet." nerdfitness.com, Nerd Fitness. October 4, 2010. Web.

"A Brief History of Southern Food." *southernfood.com*. Web.

Campbell, T. Colin, and Thomas M. Campbell II. *The China Study: Startling Implications for Diet, Weight Loss and Long-term Health*. Dallas: BenBella Books, 2006. Print.

"The Characteristics of Mediterranean Cuisine: An Overview of Typical Mediterranean Fare." *cooking-recipes-food.com*, Cooking Recipes Food. Web.

Chaudhary, Kulreet. "The Ayurvedic Diet: Eating for Your Body Type." *doctoroz.com*, The Dr. Oz Show. February 28, 2012. Web.

Chopra, Deepak. "What Is Ayurveda?" *chopra.com*, Chopra Centered Lifestyle. March 16, 2013. Web.

"Cuisine of the United States." *wikipedia.org*. Web.

Dobkin, Kelly. "What Does 'New American Cuisine' Really Mean Today?" *kerryheffernan.com*, Zagat. Web.

Editor. "If the Paleo Diet Is So Good, Why Did Cavemen Die So Young? A Look at the Pros and Cons." *livinggreenmag.com*, Living Green Magazine. October 3, 2013. Web.

English, Nick. "12 Complete Proteins vegetarians Need to Know About." *greatist.com*, Greatist. April 29, 2014. Web.

Essid, Mohamad Yassine. "Chapter 2. History of Mediterranean Food." *cairn.info*. 2012. Web.

Forks over Knives. Dir. Lee Fulkerson. Virgil Films & Entertainment (video), May 6, 2011 (in US). Film.

"The Gluten-Free Diet Plan." doctoroz.com, The Dr. Oz Show. March 22, 2011. Web

Haupt, Angela. "Raw Food Diet Overview." *usnews.com*, US News. December 12, 2013, Web.

"The Healing Properties of Juicing." *doctoroz.com*, The Dr. Oz Show. Web.

Hiatt, Kurtis. "Vegetarian Diet Overview." *usnews.com*, US News. December 13, 2013, Web.

Katz, David. "The Raw Food Diet, Overcooked." *huffingtonpost.com*, Huffpost Healthy Living. October 25, 2012. Web.

Mayo Clinic Staff. "Gluten-free Diet: What's Allowed, What's Not." *mayoclinic.org*, Mayo Clinic. Web.

Mayo Clinic Staff. "Vegetarian Diet: How to Get the best Nutrition." *mayoclinic.org*, Mayo Clinic. Web.

"Paleo Diet Overview." *usnews.com*, US News. Web.

Parker-Pope, Tara. "Confusion about Mediterranean Food." *well.blogs.nytimes.com*, The New York Times. February 11, 2009. Web.

Parker-Pope, Tara. "Nutrition Advice from the China Study." *well.blogs.nytimes.com*, The New York Times. January 7, 2011. Web.

"Raw Foods Diet." *webmd.com*, Web MD. Web.

"Starting a Raw Food Diet." *thebestofrawfood.com*, The Best of Raw Food. Web.

"10 Juicing Tips You Need to Know to Have a Highly Successful Fruit Juicing and Vegetable Juicing Program!" *holistic-medicine-works.com*, Holistic Medicine Works! Web.

thechinastudy.com

thepaleodiet.com

"Traditional Med Diet." *oldwayspt.org*, Oldways Health Through Heritage. Web.

ultimatepaleoguide.com

"Veganism in a Nutshell." *vrg.org*, The Vegetarian Resource Group. Web.

"Vegetarianism." *wikipedia.org*. Web.

Whitcomb, Amelia. "An Introduction to Mediterranean Cuisine." *lasvegasrestaurants.com*. October 16, 2008. Web.

Wolf, Robb. "The Paleo Diet Works!" *robbwolf.com*, Robb Wolf: Revolutionary Solutions f=to Modern Life. Web.

Chapter Seven - *What have You Tried in the Past?*

Agatston, Arthur. *The South Beach Diet: The Delicious, Doctor-Designed, Foolproof Plan for Fast and Healthy Weight Loss.* Rodale Books, April 5, 2003. Print.

Agatston, Arthur. *The South Beach Diet Supercharged: Faster Weight Loss and Better Health for Life.* Rodale Books, April 28, 2008, Print.

Atkins, Robert C. *Dr. Atkins' New Diet Revolution.* M. Evans & Company, July 29, 2002 (Revised Edition). Print.

atkins.com

Cruise, Jorge. *The 100: Count Only Sugar Calories and Lose Up to 18 Lbs. in 2 Weeks.* William Morrow, May 21, 2013. Print.

doctoriansmith.com

jennycraig.com

jorgecruise.com

medifast1.com

slimfast.com

Smith, Ian K. *Shred: The Revolutionary Diet: 6 Weeks 4 Inches 2 Sizes.* St. Martin's Press, December 24, 2012. Print.

southbeachdiet.com

the100diet.com

weightwatchers.com

Westman, Eric C., Stephen D. Phinney, and Jeff F. Volek. *New Atkins for a New You: The Ultimate Diet for Shedding Weight and Feeling Great*. Fireside, 2010. Print.